Basic Biomechanics

Basic Biomechanics

Maxine Durham

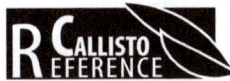

RC CALLISTO REFERENCE

www.callistoreference.com

Callisto Reference,
118-35 Queens Blvd., Suite 400,
Forest Hills, NY 11375, USA

Visit us on the World Wide Web at:
www.callistoreference.com

ISBN: 978-1-64116-632-4 (Hardback)

Cataloging-in-Publication Data

Basic biomechanics / Maxine Durham.
    p. cm.
Includes bibliographical references and index.
ISBN 978-1-64116-632-4
1. Biomechanics. 2. Contractility (Biology). 3. Biophysics. 4. Mechanics. I. Durham, Maxine.
QH513 .B37 2022
571.43--dc23

Table of Contents

Preface

The purpose of this book is to help students understand the fundamental concepts of this discipline. It is designed to motivate students to learn and prosper. I am grateful for the support of my colleagues. I would also like to acknowledge the encouragement of my family.

The study of the function, structure and motion of the mechanical aspects of biological systems by using the methods of mechanics is known as biomechanics. It is a broad field which can be divided into various sub-fields such as biofluid mechanics, biotribology, comparative biomechanics, computational biomechanics, continuum biomechanics, plant biomechanics and sports biomechanics. It ranges from the study of the inner working of a cell to the movement and development of limbs. Biomechanics also studies the mechanical properties of soft tissues, and bones. It is used in various other areas including orthopedic industry, as well as in the study of human musculoskeletal system. This book aims to shed light on some of the unexplored aspects of biomechanics. Also included herein is a detailed explanation of the various concepts and applications of biomechanics. The book is appropriate for those seeking detailed information in this area.

A foreword for all the chapters is provided below:

Chapter – What is Biomechanics?

Biomechanics is the branch of biophysics that studies the structure, function and motion of the mechanical aspects of biological systems of living organisms and their organs and cells. This chapter has been carefully written to provide an easy understanding of biomechanics.

Chapter – The Musculoskeletal System

The musculoskeletal system refers to the muscular and skeletal systems which provide form, support, stability, and movement to the body. It includes neuromuscular system, connective tissues, etc. The topics elaborated in this chapter will help in gaining a better perspective about the musculoskeletal system as well as biomechanics of its injuries.

Chapter – Concepts in Biomechanics

Some of the concepts of biomechanics include aggregate modulus, limits of stability, ground reaction force, Hill's muscle model, Moens-Korteweg equation, gait cycle, functional spinal unit, Womersley number, Tinetti test, etc. This chapter closely examines these key concepts of biomechanics to provide an extensive understanding of the subject.

Chapter – Tissue Biomechanics

Tissue biomechanics deals with the study of functions of bone, tendons and muscles to an external force. The mechanical causes of damage on these tissues are also studied within this field. This chapter has been carefully written to provide an easy understanding of tissue biomechanics.

Chapter – Locomotion

Locomotion is the movement of an organism from one place to another. Animal locomotion, bird flight, insect flight, aquatic locomotion, etc. fall under the study of locomotion. This chapter delves into the subject of locomotion to provide an in-depth understanding of it.

Chapter – Subfields of Biomechanics

The subfields of biomechanics include sports biomechanics, computational biomechanics, biofluid dynamics, nanobiomechanics, neuro biomechanics, kinesiology, biomechatronics, biotribology, etc. All these subfields of biomechanics have been carefully analyzed in this chapter.

Maxine Durham

1

What is Biomechanics?

Biomechanics is the branch of biophysics that studies the structure, function and motion of the mechanical aspects of biological systems of living organisms and their organs and cells. This chapter has been carefully written to provide an easy understanding of biomechanics.

Biomechanics is the study of biological systems, particularly their structure and function, using methods derived from mechanics, which is concerned with the effects that forces have on the motion of bodies. Ideas and investigations relating to biomechanics date back at least to the Renaissance, when Italian physiologist and physicist Giovanni Alfonso Borelli first described the basis of muscular and skeletal dynamics. Research in biomechanics became more widely known in the 20th century.

Contemporary biomechanics is a multidisciplinary field that combines physical and engineering expertise with knowledge from the biological and medical sciences. There are multiple specialty areas in biomechanics, such as cardiovascular biomechanics, cell biomechanics, human movement biomechanics (in particular orthopedic biomechanics), occupational biomechanics, and sport biomechanics. As an example, sport biomechanics deals with performance improvement and injury prevention in athletes. In occupational biomechanics, biomechanical analysis is used to understand and optimize mechanical interaction of workers with the environment.

Biomechanics research has fueled a diverse range of advances, many of which affect daily human life. Development of the biomechanics of labour, for example, focused on increasing worker efficiency without sacrificing labour safety. It resulted in the design of new tools, furniture, and other elements of a working environment that minimize load on the worker's body. Another development was clinical biomechanics, which employs mechanical facts, methodologies, and mathematics to interpret and analyze typical and atypical human anatomy and physiology.

During World War I and World War II, there was significant focus on the development of prosthetic limbs for amputee veterans, which led to major progress in biomechanics and rehabilitation medicine. Work in that area focused on increasing the mechanical efficiency of orthopedic implants, such as those used for hip or knee replacements. A biomechanics research-based approach also helped contribute to improvements in walking devices designed for individuals with lower-leg amputation and children with cerebral palsy. The development of a new class of prosthetic feet that store and return mechanical energy during walking allowed for a reduction of metabolic expenditure in amputees and made it possible for individuals with amputation to participate in athletic activities. The biomechanically based design of assistive devices, such as wheelchairs, and the optimization of environmental elements, such as stairs, allowed individuals with disabilities to improve their mobility.

The applications of biomechanics are wide-ranging. Some examples include the use of biomechanical analysis in the design of implantable artificial prostheses, such as artificial hearts and small-diameter blood vessels; in the engineering of living tissues, such as heart valves and intervertebral discs; and in injury prevention related to vehicle accidents, including low-speed collisions involving minor soft-tissue injuries and high-speed collisions involving severe and fatal injuries.

Elements

- Statics: Studying systems that are in equilibrium, either at rest or moving at a constant velocity.

- Dynamics: Studying systems that are in motion with acceleration and deceleration.

- Kinematics: Describing the effect of forces on a system, motion patterns including linear and angular changes in velocity over time. Position, displacement, velocity, and acceleration are studied.

- Kinetics: Studying what causes motion, the forces and moments at work.

Spine Biomechanics

To understand the motion of the spine and how it supports movement, we must first understand each component and the overall structure of the spine. The spine serves as a structural column providing the human body physical durability and protection. There are 32–34 total bones in the spine, divided into 5 regions: 7 vertebrae in the cervical region, 12 in the thoracic region, 5 in the lumbar region, 5 in the sacral region, and 3–5 in the coccygeal region. In between these spinal bones, there are 23 discs. The bones and discs, in combination with muscles and ligaments, allow the lumbar, thoracic, and cervical spine, different degrees of mobility. This is measured through rotational, side to side, and front to back bending. As mobile humans, it is important to realize the impact of certain activities on the spine, in order to avoid injuries and spinal conditions. Looking at the spine as a purely mechanical system, solutions can be identified using engineering principles. By making use of medical professionals' expertise in surgical procedures and the human body and engineers expertise in mechanical systems and hardware, spinal disorders can be treated. The motion of the spine is very complex, and in order to fully understand the biomechanics of this system, the components, motion, force transmission, conditions, and treatment of the spine must be examined. Understanding the motion of the spine and how it supports movement eases the understanding of each component and the overall structure of the spine. The spine serves as a structural column providing the human body physical durability and protection. The bones and discs, in combination with muscles and ligaments, allow the lumbar, thoracic, and cervical spine to move with different degrees of mobility. This is measured through rotational and lateral bending and flexion/extension. The motion of the spine is complex. By fully understanding the biomechanics of the spine as a mechanical system, the components, motion, force transmission, and conditions of the spine can be harnessed to develop new technologies in vibration reduction, sports performance, and new methods and practices for spinal surgery.

Articular Cartilage Biomechanics

Cartilage is an essential component of the human body. It plays multiple roles throughout the body, and without it our bodies would not have the ability to respond to the demanding nature of our everyday lives. Cartilage is the basis of skeletal growth; it transmits and cushions demanding loads throughout brittle bone structures. Also, it gives elasticity and shape to surrounding tissues, all this while being an avascular tissue. The complexity of cartilage's biomechanical behavior makes cartilage a demanding field of research within the biomedical engineering industry. There is ample information in the literature on the three different types of cartilage: hyaline, fibro, and elastic cartilage. Studies of the composition of articular cartilage concluded that the ECM is made up of collagen, proteoglycans, chondrocytes, and water. Collagen is the main structure in the extracellular space, while proteoglycans are heavily glycosylated proteins with a core protein with one or more covalently attached sugar chains. Chondrocytes are the single existing cell within the articular cartilage and are highly specialized and metabolically active while water is the most abundant component contributing to approximately 80% of the wet weight. Further research into the structure of articular cartilage (AC) found four distinct zones, including superficial, middle, deep, and calcified; all of which have distinct differences in composition. Within these four zones, three regions are present referenced as the territorial, pericellular, and interterritorial region. Initiating signal transduction throughout the loaded cartilage between chondrocytes and the ECM is controlled by the territorial region, which also surrounds the pericellular region. Bundles of large collagen fibers that are randomly oriented and have varying proteoglycans define the interterritorial region. Articular cartilage was found to be biphasic and anisotropic giving it distinctly different tensile and compressive properties. The viscoelastic nature of AC is also governed by its liquid and solid ECM phases leading to creep and stress relaxation behavior. Boundary layer lubrication transitioning to fluid film lubrication yields the very low coefficient of friction required to prevent cartilage deterioration between joints. Mechanical materials available today do not present the combination of elasticity and strength articular cartilage possesses making medical replacements less than ideal.

Finally, medical conditions and treatments were covered including osteoarthritis, microfracture, osteotomy, arthroplasty, stem cell therapy, and hydrogels. Current treatments do provide some alleviation of pain and discomfort; however, high costs and unwanted growth of fibro instead of hyaline cartilage leave room for further improvement in this area of the biomedical industry.

Biomechanics of Atherosclerosis

Currently, atherosclerosis is the leading cause of deaths in the developed world. Due to the nature of this disease and how prevalent it is in our modern society, it is important for all to understand how this disease manifests and is detected, as well as how it can be prevented. Atherosclerosis is a silent killer and contributes to many deaths throughout the world every year. It develops over a long period of time due to a buildup of LDL on the arterial wall before the body contains it with a mesh of collagen and elastin fibers called a fibrous cap. Based on the volume that the soft plaque occupies and the thickness of the fibrous cap itself, a person can live for years without that plaque being a danger to their health. The issue arises when the necrotic core takes up 40% or more of the volume of the plaque or if the fibrous cap is less than 65 μm thick. If either of these criteria are met, the plaque is at risk of rupturing and creating a thrombus that will kill the victim. Even without rupturing, the stiffening of the arterial wall leads to physical changes in the body's function. These changes include increased shear stress in the blood vessels, changes in systolic and diastolic blood pressures, and increased pressure fluctuations in the arteries. Thankfully in our modern age, atherosclerotic plaques can be detected and treated through a variety of methods. Each method has its advantages and disadvantages. Certain procedures excel at identifying atherosclerosis in certain arteries but struggle in other arteries. For these reasons, multiple procedures can be used together to allow a better picture of the health of a patient's arteries. It is becoming more common to use noninvasive procedures as they become more advanced. In many cases, they are just as effective as invasive procedures at detecting atherosclerosis. As atherosclerosis becomes more common, research on the disease is expanding. Every year, doctors are becoming more equipped to handle atherosclerosis.

Knee Joint Biomechanics

During everyday activities like walking and climbing up stairs, the knee experiences 2.7–4.9 times the body weight. It is a wonder how the knee can withstand so much weight over such a long period of time. Millions of years of evolution and adaptation can be found in the knee as it seems to be built for exactly what humans need it to do. The knee is meant to bear load and help the body move at the same time, and it does just that. The meniscus not only reduces the friction between our femur and tibia but also reduces the stress felt on the tibia. Humans often stand for longer periods of time, and the knee has a mechanism to reduce the amount of force needed to stay standing upright. More recently in the field of biomedical engineering, procedures are being developed to fix the issues caused by trauma or simply by degradation.

Muscle Biomechanics

Muscle is a complex tissue that is involved in many processes and systems essential to human life. They are used for balance, stability, movement, organ function, lifting objects, and many other things. This tissue needs to be analyzed from the smallest unit all the way up to the macroscale of its involvement in complex functions. Furthermore, certain engineering applications and considerations needs to be covered. Through analysis of fundamental structures and functions, the role of the muscle in the body needs to be explored, and its relevance to human life needs to be discussed. Muscle is a contractile tissue within the body responsible for internal and external locomotion and posture. There are different types of muscle tissue, composed of different types of fibers. Contractions are stimulated by the nervous system and have a specific need for energy depending on their environment. In addition, adaptations to the structure and function will arise when exposed to stimuli such as exercise. Muscle is a complex, versatile tissue which provides humans with the ability to execute a variety of tasks. The interactions of muscle tissue with the rest of the body perform many different functions that need to be carried out simply and effectively. From the contraction of single muscle fibers all the way to the entire muscle groups working together to complete a movement, the structure and fundamental properties of muscles work cooperatively to fulfill different functions and needs of the body.

Vascular Grafts

Proper circulation of blood throughout the body is extremely crucial to a long and healthy life. Any infliction that inhibits the normal flow of blood through the vast network of blood vessels poses an extreme risk to patients and can cause numerous potentially fatal conditions depending on their location. Vascular grafts are a surgical method utilized to redirect blood flow from one area to another whether to bypass a clogged or narrowed blood vessel or provide an easy access point for other procedures such as blood dialysis. It is an unfortunate truth that, in their current state, synthetic grafts are not a long-term solution to vascular stenosis and provide only small extensions on expected life spans. With the current state of undesirable compliance mismatch that exists between them and the vessels that they are grafted too, it is clear that there is a lot of room for improvement. Future research on the use of multicomponent synthetic grafts in which multiple materials are used together to better mimic the elastin and collagen mechanical properties of natural arteries and veins has a potential for improving the compliance of synthetic grafts, which ultimately leads to improved patency over time. As for tissue engineering, it is being constantly improved upon every single day. The future of biomedical engineering lays in the replication of human tissues through tissue engineering. The only way to correctly mimic the compliance of a human blood vessel is to use a form of tissue engineering. Many improvements have been made already, with some very promising results as seen in the hybrid scaffold methods as well as the decellularized matrices. It is important to note that the highest potential lies in the assembly processes. These are the processes that will allow for any mechanical property and shape to be designed exactly. The only limiting factor being the excessive amount of time required in order to manufacture these grafts. Finally the research toward sutures and the anastomotic site is also a very key area. With the hypercompliant zone being so detrimental, it is very important to consider alternate forms of sutures to combat the high compliance mismatch of those areas. In the future it can be said that a form of biocompatible glue or laser or even a combination of both may be the best choice of suture. In order for this to happen a lot of work needs to be done in those areas in order to formulate techniques in which the negatives previously mentioned are mitigated.

Transcatheter Heart Valves

Severe aortic stenosis is the calcification of the aortic heart valve that affects 3% of the world's population over the age of 75. This disease may have a variety of causes, such as age, gender, hyperlipidemia, rheumatic fever, hypertension, heart infection, abnormal stresses, and congenital abnormalities. Due to the extremely invasive nature of open-heart surgery, the mortality rate for older patients is very high, and until 1992 these patients would have had to take the risk of open-heart surgery or have no treatment and left to endure cardiac failure. Henning Rud Andersen invented an alternative surgery to replace the native aortic valve, known as a transcatheter aortic valve replacement (TAVR), also known as a percutaneous aortic valve replacement (PAVR). This surgery is done by using various catheters and medical imaging machines to allow for a replacement valve to be directed up an artery to the diseased native aortic valve. The catheter is most commonly inserted into the iliac artery or femoral artery, but there are other methods surgeons use based on their patient. A sheath is placed in an incision located near the groin to aid in inserting various surgical tools and the replacement valve into the artery. A flexible guide wire is transported to the valve to guide the surgical tools and new valve to the native valve. The native valve is then crushed using a procedure called aortic balloon valvuloplasty. Doctors will often use a method called fast pacing during an aortic balloon valvuloplasty to reduce the pulsatile aortic flow by increasing the heart rate to approximately 200 beats/min or greater. After crushing the native valve, a new bioprosthetic aortic valve is set in place using either a balloon expandable PAV or a self-expanding PAV. Doctors use various medical imaging techniques such as fluoroscopy, aortography, and echocardiography in the procedure to monitor flow characteristics and valve deployment location. This procedure is far less invasive than open-heart surgery and gives a safe alternative for older patients or patients characterized with a high mortality rate to receive a new aortic valve. The percutaneous valve is still a growing technology and is still in its optimizing stage. Issues with the valve include thrombosis (blood clotting), valve migration (due to the valve not being sutured in), stent malposition (due to physician error or valve migration), coronary obstruction, and issues with the catheter-based delivery and valve durability. Research into correcting these issues is essential for further optimizing the current models of the percutaneous heart valve and for minimizing negative inoperative and postoperative implications.

2

The Musculoskeletal System

The musculoskeletal system refers to the muscular and skeletal systems which provide form, support, stability, and movement to the body. It includes neuromuscular system, connective tissues, etc. The topics elaborated in this chapter will help in gaining a better perspective about the musculoskeletal system as well as biomechanics of its injuries.

The musculoskeletal system is an organ system that enables an organism to move, support itself, and maintain stability during locomotion.

The musculoskeletal system (also known as the locomotor system) is an organ system that gives animals (including humans) the ability to move, using the muscular and skeletal systems. It provides form, support, stability, and movement to the body.

The musculoskeletal system is made up of the body's bones (the skeleton), muscles, cartilage, tendons, ligaments, joints, and other connective tissue that supports and binds tissues and organs together.

Its primary functions include supporting the body, allowing motion, and protecting vital organs. The bones of the skeletal system provide stability to the body analogous to a reinforcement bar in concrete construction.

Muscles keep bones in place and also play a role in their movement. To allow motion, different bones are connected by articulating joints, and cartilage prevents the bone ends from rubbing directly onto each other.

Skeletal System

The skeletal portion of the system serves as the main storage system for calcium and phosphorus. The importance of this storage is to help regulate mineral balance in the bloodstream. When the fluctuation of minerals is high, these minerals are stored in bone; when it is low, minerals are withdrawn from the bone.

The skeleton also contains critical components of the hematopoietic (blood production) system. Located in long bones are two distinctions of bone marrow: yellow and red. The yellow marrow has fatty connective tissue and is found in the marrow cavity. In times of starvation, the body uses the fat in yellow marrow for energy.

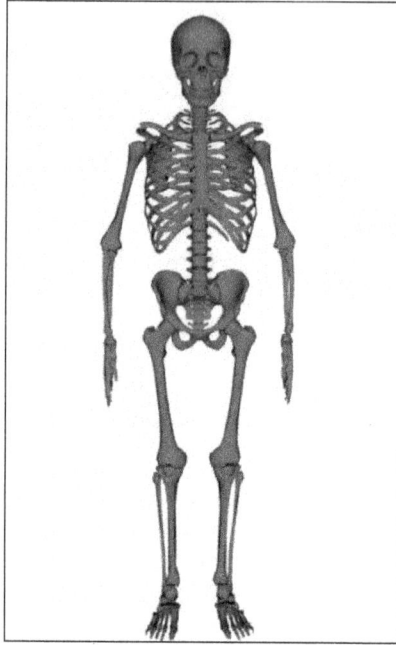

A human skeleton: Image as overview of the human skeletal system.

The red marrow of some bones is an important site for hematopoeisis or blood cell production that replaces cells that have been destroyed by the liver. Here, all erythrocytes, platelets, and most leukocytes form in bone marrow from where they migrate to the circulation.

Muscular System

Muscles contract (shorten) to move the bone attached at the joint. Skeletal muscles are attached to bones and arranged in opposing groups around joints. Muscles are innervated—the nerves conduct electrical currents from the central nervous system that cause the muscles to contract.

Three types of muscle tissue exist in the body. These are skeletal, smooth, and cardiac muscle.

- Only skeletal and smooth muscles are considered part of the musculoskeletal system.

- Skeletal m uscle is involved in body locomotion.

- Examples of smooth muscles include those found in intestinal and vessel walls.

- Cardiac and smooth muscle are characterized by involuntary movement (not under conscious control).

- Cardiac muscles are found in the heart.

Tendons, Joints, Ligaments and Bursae

A tendon is a tough, flexible band made of fibrous connective tissue, and functions to connect muscle to bone. Joints are the bone articulations allowing movement. A ligament is a dense, white band of fibrous elastic tissue.

Ligaments connect the ends of bones together in order to form a joint. These help to limit joint dislocation and restrict improper hyperextension and hyperflexion. Also made of fibrous tissue are bursae. These provide cushions between bones and tendons and/or muscles around a joint.

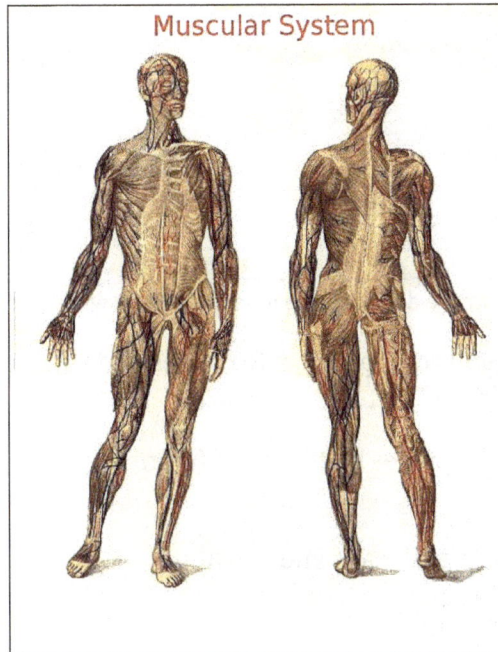

Musculoskeletal system: Image depicting the human muscular system (skeletal muscle).

The Axial Skeleton

The axial skeleton functions to support and protect the organs of the dorsal and ventral cavities and serves as a surface for the attachment of muscles and parts of the appendicular skeleton.

The axial skeleton is the part of the skeleton that consists of the bones of the head and trunk of a vertebrate animal, including humans.

The word axial is from the word axis, and refers to how the bones of the axial skeleton are located along the central axis of the body.

The axial skeleton functions to support and protect the organs of the dorsal and ventral cavities. It also serves as a surface for the attachment of muscles and parts of the appendicular skeleton.

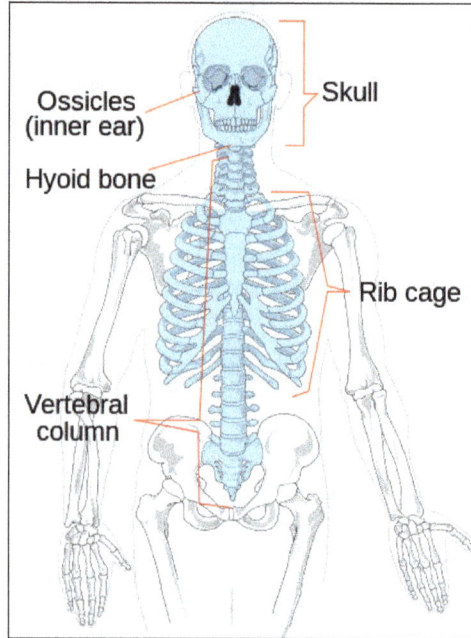

Axial skeleton: Image depicting the human skeleton with the axial skeleton.

The human's axial skeleton is composed of 80 bones and is the central core of the body. The primary divisions of the skeleton system are:

- Head, including the bones of the skull (cranium), face, auditory ossicles, and hyoid bone.

- Thorax, including the rib cage and sternum.

- Vertebral column.

Bones of the Head

Skull (Cranium)

The human cranium consists of the flat bones of the cranium and includes the facial bones. The cranium protects the brain that is contained in the cranial vault. The cranium is formed from eight bones connected by sutures.

Fourteen facial bones form the lower front part of the cranium. Important facial bones include the lower jaw or mandible, the upper jaw or maxilla, the zygomatic or cheek bone, and the nasal bone.

The immature cranium has separate plates to allow the flexibility needed for a newborn to pass through the birth canal and pelvis.

These plates fuse as the skull matures (except the mandible). The human cranium supports the structures of the face and forms the brain cavity.

Ossicle

The ossicles (also called auditory ossicles) consist of three bones (malleus, incus, and stapes) that are the smallest in the body. These are located in the middle ear and serve to transmit sounds from the air to the fluid-filled labyrinth.

Hyoid Bone

The hyoid bone is a horseshoe-shaped bone situated in the anterior midline of the neck between the chin and the thyroid cartilage. It provides attachment to the muscles of the floor of the mouth, the tongue above, larynx below, and the epiglottis and pharynx behind.

Rib Cage

The rib cage is composed of 25 bones that include the 12 pairs of ribs plus the sternum. It functions as protection for the vital organs of the chest, such as the heart and lungs. The rounded ends are attached at joints to the thoracic vertebrae posteriorly and the flattened ends come together at the sternum anteriorly.

The first seven pairs of ribs attach to the sternum with costal cartilage and are known as true ribs. Thelength of each rib pair increases from number one to seven. After rib seven, the size begins to decrease. The 8th through 10th ribs have noncostal cartilage that connects them to the ribs above.

The last two ribs are called floating ribs because they do not attach to the sternum or to other ribs.

Vertebral Column

There are normally thirty-three vertebrae in the human vertebral column. The upper twenty-four articulate and are unfused, the lower nine are fused. The fused vertebrae are the five in the sacrum and four in the coccyx.

The articulating vertebrae are named according regions:

- Cervical vertebrae (seven vertebrae).
- Thoracic (twelve vertebrae).
- Lumbar (five vertebrae).

The first and second cervical vertebrae are the atlas and axis, respectively, on which the head rests. The cervical vertebrae make up the junction between the vertebral column and the cranium, and the bone makes up the junction between the vertebral column and the pelvic bones.

The Appendicular Skeleton

The appendicular skeleton includes the skeletal elements within the limbs, as well as supporting pectoral and pelvic girdles.

The appendicular skeleton of vertebrates, including humans, consists of the bones that support and compose the appendages (for example, the arms and legs of humans). The word appendicular is the adjective of the noun appendage.

The appendicular skeleton includes the skeletal elements within the limbs, as well as supporting the pectoral and pelvic girdles.

The appendicular skeleton comprises 126 bones and is involved in locomotion and manipulation of objects in the environment. It is unfused, allowing for greater range of motion.

Divisions of the Appendicular Skeleton

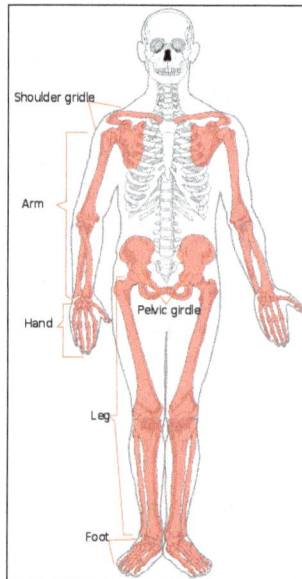

A diagram of the apendicular skeleton: Image depicting the human skeleton with the appendicular skeleton colored red.

The appendicular skeleton is divided into six major regions:

- The pectoral girdles consist of 4 bones: The left and right clavicle (2) and the scapula (2).

- The upper arms and forearms are made up of 6 bones: The left and right humerus (upper arm, 2), the ulna (2), and the radius (forearm, 2).

- The hands have 54 bones: The left and right carpals (wrist, 16), metacarpals (10), proximal phalanges (10), intermediate phalanges (8), and the distal phalanges (10).

- The pelvis has 2 bones: The left and right hip bone (2).

- The thighs and legs have 8 bones: The left and right femur (thigh, 2), patella (knee, 2), tibia (2) and fibula (leg, 2).

- The feet and ankles have 52 bones: The left and right tarsals (ankle, 14), metatarsals (10), proximal phalanges (10), intermediate phalanges (8), and distal phalanges (10).

Pectoral Girdle

The bones of the pectoral girdle consist of two bones (scapula and clavicle) and anchor the upper limb to the thoracic cage of the axial skeleton.

The three regions of the upper limb are: arm (humerus), forearm (ulna medially and radius laterally), and the hand.

The base of the hand contains eight bones (carpal bones), and the palm is formed by five bones (metacarpal bones). The fingers and thumb contain a total of 14 bones, called phalanges.

Pelvic Girdle

The pelvic girdle is formed by a single bone, the hip or coxal bone, and serves as the attachment point for each lower limb. Each hip bone is joined to the axial skeleton by its attachment to the sacrum of the vertebral column. The right and left hip bones attach to each other anteriorly.

The lower limb contains 30 bones and is divided into three regions, the thigh, leg, and foot. These consist of the femur, patella, tibia, fibula, tarsal bones, metatarsal bones, and phalanges.

- The femur is the single bone of the thigh.

- The patella (kneecap) articulates with the distal femur.

- The tibia is located on the medial side of the leg,

- The fibula is the thin bone of the lateral leg.

The bones of the foot are divided into three groups, the tarsal bones, metatarsal bones, and phalanges of the foot.

SKELETON

The skeleton is the body part that forms the supporting structure of an organism. It can also be seen as the bony frame work of the body which provides support, shape and protection to the soft tissues and delicate organs in animals. There are several different skeletal types: the exoskeleton, which is the stable outer shell of an organism, the endoskeleton, which forms the support structure inside the body, the hydroskeleton, a flexible skeleton supported by fluid pressure, and the cytoskeleton present in the cytoplasm of all cells, including bacteria, and archaea.

Types of Skeletons

There are two major types of skeletons: solid and fluid. Solid skeletons can be internal, called an endoskeleton, or external, called an exoskeleton, and may be further classified as pliant (elastic/movable) or rigid (hard/non-movable).

Exoskeleton

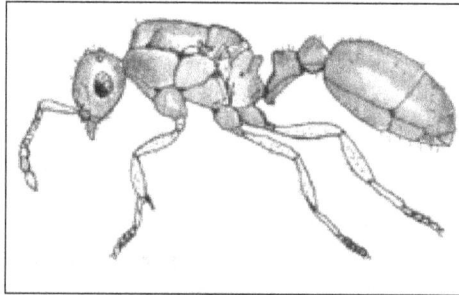

Exoskeleton of an ant.

Exoskeletons are external, and are found in many invertebrates; they enclose and protect the soft tissues and organs of the body. Some kinds of exoskeletons undergo periodic moulting or ecdysis as the animal grows, as is the case in many arthropods including insects and crustaceans.

The exoskeleton of insects is not only a form of protection, but also serves as a surface for muscle attachment, as a watertight protection against drying, and as a sense organ to interact with the environment. The shell of mollusks also performs all of the same functions, except that in most cases it does not contain sense organs.

An external skeleton can be quite heavy in relation to the overall mass of an animal, so on land, organisms that have an exoskeleton are mostly relatively small. Somewhat larger aquatic animals can support an exoskeleton because weight is less of a consideration underwater. The southern giant clam, a species of extremely large saltwater clam in the Pacific Ocean, has a shell that is massive in both size and weight. Syrinx aruanus is a species of sea snail with a very large shell.

Endoskeleton

The endoskeleton is the internal support structure of an animal, composed of mineralized tissue and is typical of vertebrates. Endoskeletons vary in complexity from functioning purely for support (as in the case of sponges), to serving as an attachment site for muscles and a mechanism for transmitting muscular forces. A true endoskeleton is derived from mesodermal tissue. Such a skeleton is present in echinoderms and chordates.

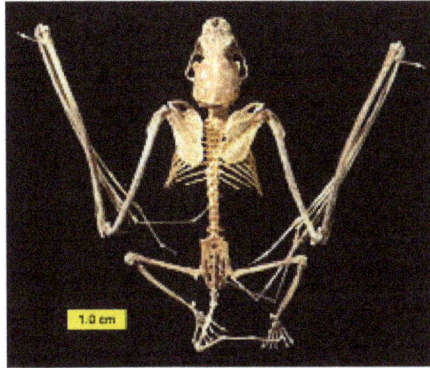

Endoskeleton of a bat.

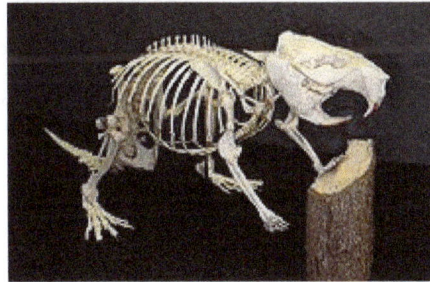

A beaver skeleton on display at The Museum of Osteology, Oklahoma City, Oklahoma.

Pliant Skeletons

Pliant skeletons are capable of movement; thus, when stress is applied to the skeletal structure, it deforms and then reverts to its original shape. This skeletal structure is used in some invertebrates, for instance in the hinge of bivalve shells or the mesoglea of cnidarians such as jellyfish. Pliant skeletons are beneficial because only muscle contractions are needed to bend the skeleton; upon muscle relaxation, the skeleton will return to its original shape. Cartilage is one material that a pliant skeleton may be composed of, but most pliant skeletons are formed from a mixture of proteins, polysaccharides, and water. For additional structure or protection, pliant skeletons may be supported by rigid skeletons. Organisms that have pliant skeletons typically live in water, which supports body structure in the absence of a rigid skeleton.

Rigid Skeletons

Rigid skeletons are not capable of movement when stressed, creating a strong support system most common in terrestrial animals. Such a skeleton type used by animals that live in water are more for protection (such as barnacle and snail shells) or for fast-moving animals that require additional support of musculature needed for swimming through water. Rigid skeletons are formed from materials including chitin (in arthropods), calcium compounds such as calcium carbonate (in stony corals and mollusks) and silicate (for diatoms and radiolarians).

Cytoskeleton

The cytoskeleton is used to stabilize and preserve the form of the cells. It is a dynamic structure that maintains cell shape, protects the cell, enables cellular motion (using structures such as flagella, cilia and lamellipodia), and plays important roles in both intracellular transport (the movement of vesicles and organelles, for example) and cellular division.

Fluid Skeletons

Hydrostatic Skeleton (Hydroskeleton)

A hydrostatic skeleton is a semi-rigid, soft tissue structure filled with liquid under pressure, surrounded by muscles. Longitudinal and circular muscles around their body sectors allow movement by alternate lengthening and contractions along their lengths. A common example of this is the earthworm.

Organisms with Skeletons

Invertebrates

The endoskeletons of echinoderms and some other soft-bodied invertebrates such as jellyfish and earthworms are also termed hydrostatic; a body cavity the coelom is filled with coelomic fluid and the pressure from this fluid acts together with the surrounding muscles to change the organism's shape and produce movement.

Sponges

The skeleton of sponges consists of microscopic calcareous or silicious spicules. The demosponges include 90% of all species of sponges. Their "skeletons" are made of spicules consisting of fibers of the protein spongin, the mineral silica, or both. Where spicules of silica are present, they have a different shape from those in the otherwise similar glass sponges.

Echinoderms

The skeleton of the echinoderms, which include, among other things, the starfish, is composed of calcite and a small amount of magnesium oxide. It lies below the epidermis in the mesoderm and is within cell clusters of frame-forming cells. This structure formed is porous and therefore firm and at the same time light. It coalesces into small calcareous ossicles (bony plates), which can grow in all directions and thus can replace the loss of a body part. Connected by joints, the individual skeletal parts can be moved by the muscles.

Vertebrates

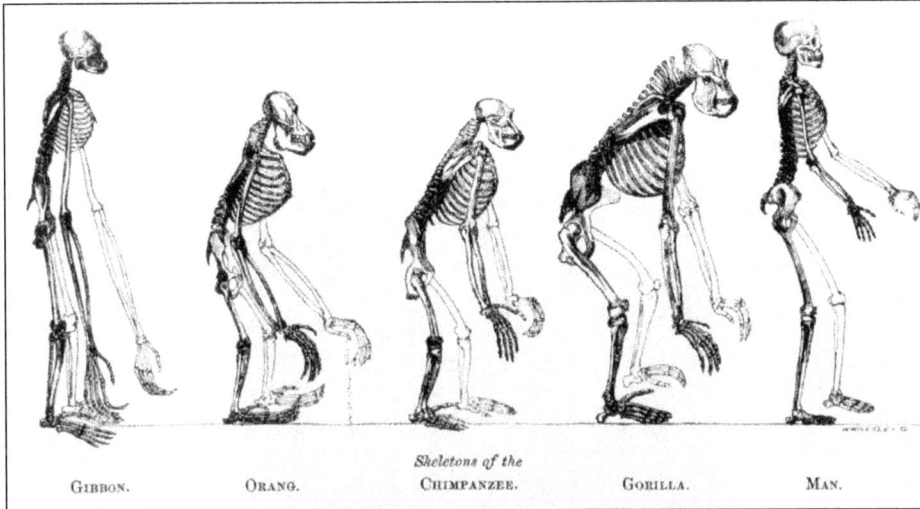

Pithecometra: From Thomas Huxley's 1863 Evidence as to Man's Place
in Nature, the compared skeletons of apes to humans.

In most vertebrates, the main skeletal component is referred to as bone. These bones compose a unique skeletal system for each type of animal. Another important component is cartilage which in mammals is found mainly in the joint areas. In other animals, such as the cartilaginous fishes, which include the sharks, the skeleton is composed entirely of cartilage. The segmental pattern of the skeleton is present in all vertebrates (mammals, birds, fish, reptiles and amphibians) with basic units being repeated. This segmental pattern is particularly evident in the vertebral column and the ribcage.

Bones in addition to supporting the body also serve, at the cellular level, as calcium and phosphate storage.

Fish

The skeleton, which forms the support structure inside the fish is either made of cartilage as in the (Chondrichthyes), or bones as in the (Osteichthyes). The main skeletal element is the vertebral column, composed of articulating vertebrae which are lightweight yet strong. The ribs attach to the spine and there are no limbs or limb girdles. They are supported only by the muscles. The main external features of the fish, the fins, are composed of either bony or soft spines called rays, which with the exception of the caudal fin (tail fin), have no direct connection with the spine. They are supported by the muscles which compose the main part of the trunk.

Birds

The bird skeleton is highly adapted for flight. It is extremely lightweight, yet still strong enough to withstand the stresses of taking off, flying, and landing. One key adaptation is the fusing of bones into single ossifications, such as the pygostyle. Because of this, birds usually have a smaller number of bones than other terrestrial vertebrates. Birds also lack teeth or even a true jaw, instead having evolved a beak, which is far more lightweight. The beaks of many baby birds have a projection called an egg tooth, which facilitates their exit from the amniotic egg.

Marine Mammals

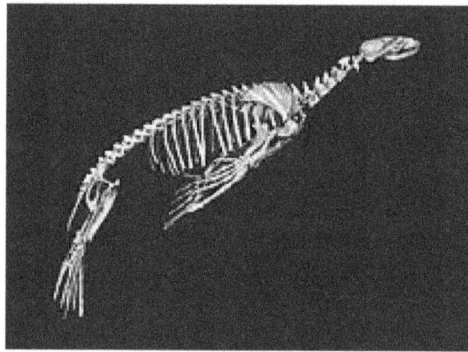

Californian sea lion.

To facilitate the movement of marine mammals in water, the hind legs were either lost altogether, as in the whales and manatees, or united in a single tail fin as in the pinnipeds (seals). In the whale, the cervical vertebrae are typically fused, an adaptation trading flexibility for stability during swimming.

Humans

The human skeleton consists of both fused and individual bones supported and supplemented by ligaments, tendons, muscles and cartilage. It serves as a scaffold which supports organs, anchors muscles, and protects organs such as the brain, lungs, heart and spinal cord. Although the teeth do not consist of tissue commonly found in bones, the teeth are usually considered as members of the skeletal system. The biggest bone in the body is the femur in the upper leg, and the smallest is the stapes bone in the middle ear. In an adult, the skeleton comprises around 14% of the total body weight, and half of this weight is water.

Fused bones include those of the pelvis and the cranium. Not all bones are interconnected directly: There are three bones in each middle ear called the ossicles that articulate only with each other. The hyoid bone, which is located in the neck and serves as the point of attachment for the tongue, does not articulate with any other bones in the body, being supported by muscles and ligaments.

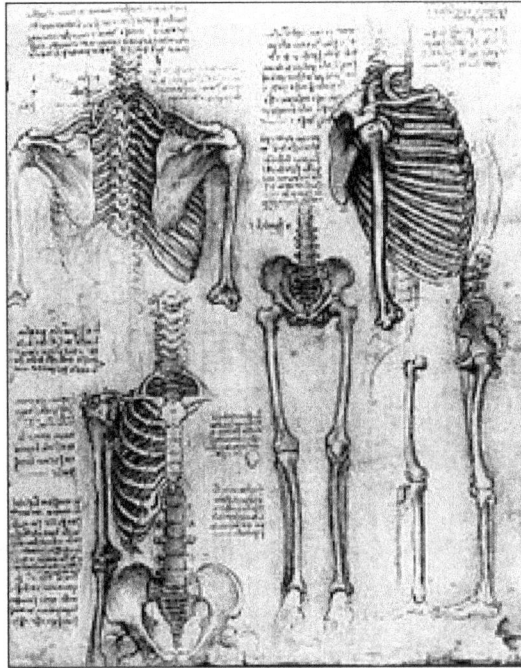

Study of Skeletons, c. 1510, by Leonardo da Vinci.

There are 206 bones in the adult human skeleton, although this number depends on whether the pelvic bones (the hip bones on each side) are counted as one or three bones on each side (ilium, ischium, and pubis), whether the coccyx or tail bone is counted as one or four separate bones, and does not count the variable wormian bones between skull sutures. Similarly, the sacrum is usually counted as a single bone, rather than five fused vertebrae. There is also a variable number of small sesamoid bones, commonly found in tendons. The patella or kneecap on each side is an example of a larger sesamoid bone. The patellae are counted in the total, as they are constant. The number of bones varies between individuals and with age – newborn babies have over 270 bones some of which fuse together. These bones are organized into a longitudinal axis, the axial skeleton, to which the appendicular skeleton is attached.

The human skeleton takes 20 years before it is fully developed. In many animals, the skeleton bones contain marrow, which produces blood cells.

There exist several general differences between the male and female skeletons. The male skeleton, for example, is generally larger and heavier than the female skeleton. In the female skeleton, the bones of the skull are generally less angular. The female skeleton also has wider and shorter breastbone and slimmer wrists. There exist significant differences between the male and female pelvis which are related to the female's pregnancy and childbirth capabilities. The female pelvis is wider and shallower than the male pelvis. Female pelvises also have an enlarged pelvic outlet and a wider and more circular pelvic inlet. The angle between the pubic bones is known to be sharper in males, which results in a more circular, narrower, and near heart-shaped pelvis.

CONNECTIVE TISSUES

Connective tissue (CT) is one of the four basic types of animal tissue, along with epithelial tissue, muscle tissue, and nervous tissue. It develops from the mesoderm. Connective tissue is found in between other tissues everywhere in the body, including the nervous system. In the central nervous system, the three outer membranes (the meninges) that envelop the brain and spinal cord are composed of connective tissue. They support and protect the body. All connective tissue consists of three main components: fibers (elastic and collagenous fibers), ground substance and cells. Not all authorities include blood or lymph as connective tissue because they lack the fiber component. All are immersed in the body water.

The cells of connective tissue include fibroblasts, adipocytes, macrophages, mast cells and leucocytes.

The term "connective tissue" (in German, Bindegewebe) was introduced in 1830 by Johannes Peter Müller. The tissue was already recognized as a distinct class in the 18th century.

Types

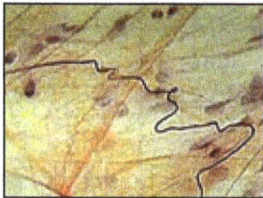
Areolar connective tissue

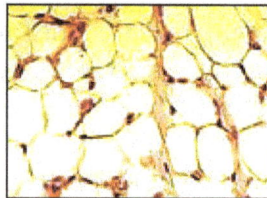
Adipose tissue

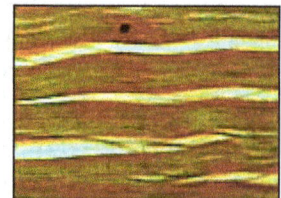
Fibrous connective tissue

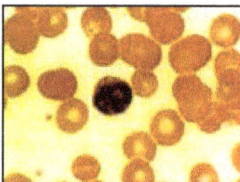
Blood

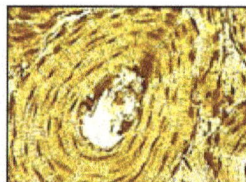
Osseous tissue

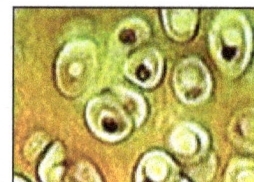
Hyaline cartilage

Connective tissue can be broadly subdivided into connective tissue proper, and special connective tissue. Connective tissue proper consists of loose connective tissue and dense connective tissue (which is further subdivided into dense regular and dense irregular connective tissues.) Loose and dense connective tissue are distinguished by the ratio of ground substance to fibrous tissue. Loose connective tissue has much more ground substance and a relative lack of fibrous tissue, while the reverse is true of dense connective tissue. Dense regular connective tissue, found in structures such as tendons and ligaments, is characterized by collagen fibers arranged in an orderly parallel fashion, giving it tensile strength in one direction. Dense irregular connective tissue provides strength in multiple directions by its dense bundles of fibers arranged in all directions.

Special connective tissue consists of reticular connective tissue, adipose tissue, cartilage, bone, and blood. Other kinds of connective tissues include fibrous, elastic, and lymphoid connective tissues. Fibroareolar tissue is a mix of fibrous and areolar tissue. Fibromuscular tissue is made up of fibrous tissue and muscular tissue. New vascularised connective tissue that forms in the process of wound healing is termed granulation tissue. Fibroblasts are the cells responsible for the production of some CT.

Type I collagen is present in many forms of connective tissue, and makes up about 25% of the total protein content of the mammalian body.

Characteristics

- Cells are spread through an extracellular fluid.

- Ground substance: A clear, colorless, and viscous fluid containing glycosaminoglycans and proteoglycans to fix the body water and the collagen fibers in the intercellular spaces. Ground substance slows the spread of pathogens.

- Fibers: Not all types of CT are fibrous. Examples of non-fibrous CT include adipose tissue and blood. Adipose tissue gives "mechanical cushioning" to the body, among other functions. Although there is no dense collagen network in adipose tissue, groups of adipose cells are kept together by collagen fibers and collagen sheets in order to keep fat tissue under compression in place (for example, the sole of the foot). The matrix of blood is plasma.

- Both the ground substance and proteins (fibers) create the matrix for CT. Connective tissues are derived from the mesenchyme.

Types of Fibers

Tissue	Purpose	Components	Location
Collagenous fibers.	Bind bones and other tissues to each other.	Alpha polypeptide chains.	tendon, ligament, skin, cornea, cartilage, bone, blood vessels, gut, and intervertebral disc.
Elastic fibers.	Allow organs like arteries and lungs to recoil.	Elastic microfibril and elastin.	extracellular matrix.
Reticular fibers.	Form a scaffolding for other cells.	Type III collagen.	liver, bone marrow, and lymphatic organs.

Function

Connective tissue has a wide variety of functions that depend on the types of cells and the different classes of fibers involved. Loose and dense irregular connective tissue, formed mainly by fibroblasts and collagen fibers, have an important role in providing a medium for oxygen and nutrients to diffuse from capillaries to cells, and carbon dioxide and waste substances to diffuse from cells back into circulation. They also allow organs to resist stretching and tearing forces. Dense regular connective tissue, which forms organized structures, is a major functional component of tendons, ligaments and aponeuroses, and is also found in highly specialized organs such as the cornea. Elastic fibers, made from elastin and fibrillin, also provide resistance to stretch forces. They are found in the walls of large blood vessels and in certain ligaments, particularly in the ligamenta flava.

In hematopoietic and lymphatic tissues, reticular fibers made by reticular cells provide the stroma—or structural support—for the parenchyma—or functional part—of the organ.

Mesenchyme is a type of connective tissue found in developing organs of embryos that is capable of differentiation into all types of mature connective tissue. Another type of relatively undifferentiated connective tissue is the mucous connective tissue known as Wharton's jelly, found inside the umbilical cord.

Various types of specialized tissues and cells are classified under the spectrum of connective tissue, and are as diverse as brown and white adipose tissue, blood, cartilage and bone. Cells of the immune system, such as macrophages, mast cells, plasma cells and eosinophils are found scattered in loose connective tissue, providing the ground for starting inflammatory and immune responses upon the detection of antigens.

Clinical Significance

There are many types of connective tissue disorders, such as:

- Connective tissue neoplasms including sarcomas such as hemangiopericytoma and malignant peripheral nerve sheath tumor in nervous tissue.

- Congenital diseases include Marfan syndrome and Ehlers-Danlos Syndrome.

- Myxomatous degeneration – a pathological weakening of connective tissue.

- Mixed connective tissue disease – a disease of the autoimmune system, also undifferentiated connective tissue disease.

- Systemic lupus erythematosus (SLE) – a major autoimmune disease of connective tissue.

- Scurvy, caused by a deficiency of vitamin C which is necessary for the synthesis of collagen.

- Fibromuscular dysplasia is a disease of the blood vessels that leads to an abnormal growth in the arterial wall.

JOINT

A joint or articulation (or articular surface) is the connection made between bones in the body which link the skeletal system into a functional whole. They are constructed to allow for different degrees and types of movement. Some joints, such as the knee, elbow, and shoulder, are self-lubricating, almost frictionless, and are able to withstand compression and maintain heavy loads while still executing smooth and precise movements. Other joints such as sutures between the bones of the skull permit very little movement (only during birth) in order to protect the brain and the sense organs. The connection between a tooth and the jawbone is also called a joint, and is described as a fibrous joint known as a gomphosis. Joints are classified both structurally and functionally.

Classification

Joints are mainly classified structurally and functionally. Structural classification is determined by how the bones connect to each other, while functional classification is determined by the degree of movement between the articulating bones. In practice, there is significant overlap between the two types of classifications.

Clinical, Numerical Classification

- Monoarticular: Concerning one joint.

- Oligoarticular or pauciarticular: Concerning 2–4 joints.

- Polyarticular: Concerning 5 or more joints.

Structural Classification (Binding Tissue)

Structural classification names and divides joints according to the type of binding tissue that connects the bones to each other. There are four structural classifications of joints:

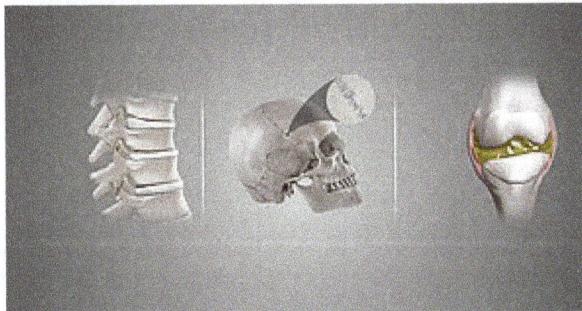

Types of joints based upon their structure (L to R): Cartilaginous joint, Fibrous joint, and Synovial joint.

- Fibrous joint: Joined by dense regular connective tissue that is rich in collagen fibers.

- Cartilaginous joint: Joined by cartilage. There are two types: primary cartilaginous joints composed of hyaline cartilage, and secondary cartilaginous joints composed of hyaline cartilage covering the articular surfaces of the involved bones with fibrocartilage connecting them.

- Synovial joint: Not directly joined – the bones have a synovial cavity and are united by the dense irregular connective tissue that forms the articular capsule that is normally associated with accessory ligaments.

- Facet joint: Joint between two articular processes between two vertebrae.

Functional Classification (Movement)

Joints can also be classified functionally according to the type and degree of movement they allow: Joint movements are described with reference to the basic anatomical planes.

- Synarthrosis: Permits little or no mobility. Most synarthrosis joints are fibrous joints (e.g., skull sutures).

- Amphiarthrosis: Permits slight mobility. Most amphiarthrosis joints are cartilaginous joints (e.g., intervertebral discs).

- Synovial joint (also known as a diarthrosis): Freely movable. Synovial joints can in turn be classified into six groups according to the type of movement they allow: plane joint, ball and socket joint, hinge joint, pivot joint, condyloid joint and saddle joint.

Joints can also be classified, according to the number of axes of movement they allow, into nonaxial (gliding, as between the proximal ends of the ulna and radius), monoaxial (uniaxial), biaxial and multiaxial. Another classification is according to the degrees of freedom allowed, and distinguished between joints with one, two or three degrees of freedom. A further classification is according to the number and shapes of the articular surfaces: flat, concave and convex surfaces. Types of articular surfaces include trochlear surfaces.

Biomechanical Classification

Joints can also be classified based on their anatomy or on their biomechanical properties. According to the anatomic classification, joints are subdivided into simple and compound, depending on the number of bones involved, and into complex and combination joints:

- Simple joint: Two articulation surfaces (e.g. shoulder joint, hip joint).

- Compound joint: Three or more articulation surfaces (e.g. radiocarpal joint).

- Complex joint: Two or more articulation surfaces and an articular disc or meniscus (e.g. knee joint).

Anatomical

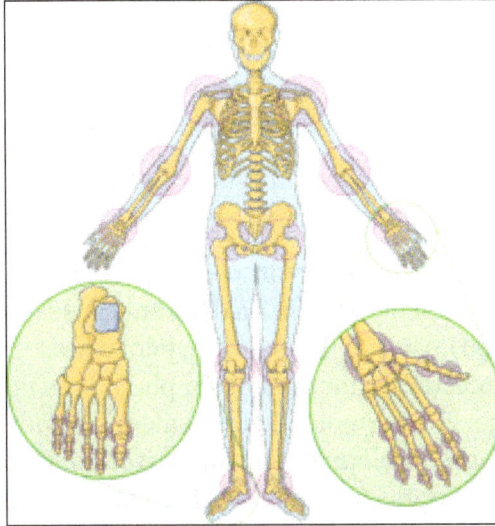

Joints of the human body.

The joints may be classified anatomically into the following groups:

- Joints of hand.

- Elbow joints.

- Wrist joints.

- Axillary articulations.

- Sternoclavicular joints.

- Vertebral articulations.

- Temporomandibular joints.

- Sacroiliac joints.

- Hip joints.

- Knee joints.

- Articulations of foot.

Unmyelinated nerve fibers are abundant in joint capsules and ligaments as well as in the outer part of intraarticular menisci. These nerve fibers are responsible for pain perception when a joint is strained.

Clinical Significance

Damaging the cartilage of joints (articular cartilage) or the bones and muscles that stabilize the joints can lead to joint dislocations and osteoarthritis. Swimming is a great way to exercise the joints with minimal damage.

A joint disorder is termed arthropathy, and when involving inflammation of one or more joints the disorder is called arthritis. Most joint disorders involve arthritis, but joint damage by external physical trauma is typically not termed arthritis.

Arthropathies are called *polyarticular* (multiarticular) when involving many joints and *monoarticular* when involving only a single joint.

Arthritis is the leading cause of disability in people over the age of 55. There are many different forms of arthritis, each of which has a different cause. The most common form of arthritis, osteoarthritis (also known as degenerative joint disease), occurs following trauma to the joint, following an infection of the joint or simply as a result of aging and the deterioration of articular cartilage. Furthermore, there is emerging evidence that abnormal anatomy may contribute to early development of osteoarthritis. Other forms of arthritis are rheumatoid arthritis and psoriatic arthritis, which are autoimmune diseases in which the body is attacking itself. Septic arthritis is caused by joint infection. Gouty arthritis is caused by deposition of uric acid crystals in the joint that results in subsequent inflammation. Additionally, there is a less common form of gout that is caused by the formation of rhomboidal-shaped crystals of calcium pyrophosphate. This form of gout is known as pseudogout.

Temporomandibular joint syndrome (TMJ) involves the jaw joints and can cause facial pain, clicking sounds in the jaw, or limitation of jaw movement, to name a few symptoms. It is caused by psychological tension and misalignment of the jaw (malocclusion), and may be affecting as many as 75 million Americans.

NEUROMUSCULAR SYSTEM

The neuromuscular system includes all the muscles in the body and the nerves serving them. Every movement your body makes requires communication between the brain and the muscles. The nervous system provides the link between thoughts and actions by relaying messages that travel so fast you don't even notice.

Nerves and muscles, working together as the neuromuscular system, make your body move as you want it to. They also make sure you do things you don't even think about, such as breathe.

Working of the Neuromuscular System

Nerves have cells called neurons. Neurons carry messages from the brain via the spinal cord. The neurons that carry these messages to the muscles are called motor neurons.

Each motor neuron ending sits very close to a muscle fibre. Where they sit together is called a neuromuscular junction. The motor neurons can release a chemical, which is picked up by the muscle fibre. This tells the muscle fibre to contract, which makes the muscles move.

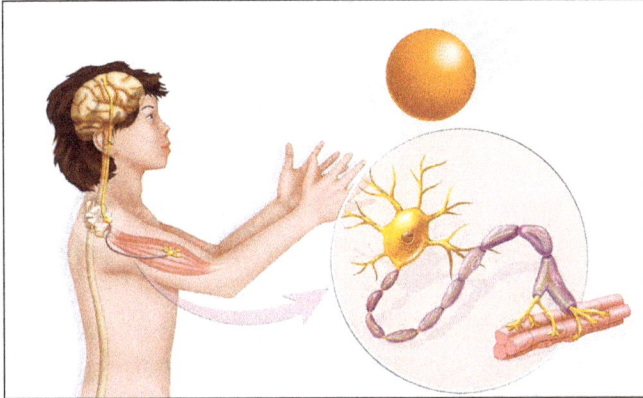

Neurons carry messages from the brain via the spinal cord. These messages are carried to the muscles which tell the muscle fibre to contract, which makes the muscles move.

Diseases Involving the Neuromuscular System

Many different diseases affect the neuromuscular system, and together they are known as neuromuscular diseases.

Some examples of neuromuscular diseases are:

- Neuropathies (problems with the nerves), such as Charcot-Marie-Tooth disease or motor neuron disease.

- Myopathies (problems with the muscles), such as muscular dystrophy.

- Neuromuscular autoimmune conditions, such as myasthenia gravis or multiple sclerosis.

In some neuromuscular diseases, the nerves are damaged, and don't carry messages from the brain as they should. In others, the muscles are damaged, and they either can't receive messages from motor neurons, or they can't respond as they should.

Either way, the person affected can have problems with tiredness, weakness, muscle pain, wasting and spasms. Often, the symptoms affect the arms and legs more than other parts of the body.

In severe cases, neuromuscular diseases can lead to difficulties in swallowing, speaking and breathing.

Treatments for neuromuscular disorders generally aim to ease symptoms and improve quality of life, but in many cases there are no effective medications. Unfortunately, most neuromuscular disorders cannot currently be cured.

MUSCULOSKELETAL INJURY

Musculoskeletal injuries result from the damage of muscular or skeletal systems, which usually occur due to a strenuous and/or repetitive activity. They are among the most common work-related injuries.

They include a number of disorders involving muscles, bones, tendons, blood vessels, nerves, and other soft tissues. Commonly referred to as repetitive strain injury (RSI), some examples of musculoskeletal disorders include carpal tunnel syndrome, tendonitis, tenosynovitis, and bursitis. Treatments vary and can produce different results. Physical or occupational therapy is sometimes used to help injured workers return to work quickly and safely with learned skills to avoid re-injury.

The traumatic injuries of the muscles, tendons, and nerves are usually a result of accidents or repetitive, straining activities. Work activities that are frequent and repetitive, or activities that require workers to adopt an awkward posture, are the most common cause of musculoskeletal injuries, which may be painful during work or at rest.

Common movements, such as bending, straightening, gripping, holding, twisting, clenching, and reaching are hazardous in work situations as their continual repetition, often in a forceful manner, is associated with the development of musculoskeletal injuries.

Biomechanics of Musculoskeletal Injury

Fracture as a result of traumatic injury is a major contributor to long-term disability and loss of work and is therefore an important health concern, as well as contributor to overall societal economic burden. A total of 1.5 million fractures occur each year, including 280,000 hip fractures and 500,000 vertebral fractures. Because the human musculoskeletal system is a living organ with predominantly a mechanical role, physiology and engineering principles are critical for its study and understanding. Fracture and musculoskeletal injury occur when local stresses or strains exceed the ultimate strength of bones, tendons, ligaments and muscles. These tissues regenerate, heal, or fail to heal according to both mechanical and biological stimuli.

Acute Injury and Inflammation

Injury occurs when local stress or strain exceed the ultimate strength of bones and soft tissue. Since all tissues are to some degree viscoelastic, the rate at which energy is dissipated also contributes to the degree of tissue injury since tissue stiffness, which often defines failure modes, is dependent on rate of deformation. Unlike most materials, living tissues also respond to a traumatic event, not only with mechanical failure, but with an acute inflammatory response. This inflammatory response results in the sudden and extended release of inflammatory mediators, cytokines, and other factors that act, not only locally to define the injury and to initiate what ultimately will be the healing response, but also may have significant systemic effects, potentially resulting in severe pulmonary injury or end stage organ failure. Inflammatory cascades are initiated, not only in traumatized tissues, but also by pathogens, or other foreign irritants. In the setting of trauma, these inflammatory mediators are intimately associated with the healing process. They attract precursors for cell growth, and they modulate repair mechanisms. Inflammation also stimulates and increases the sensitivity of pain receptors, which serve a protective purpose, causing trauma patients to limit motion around the damaged tissue.

Inflammation is an acute immune response, designed to rid the organism of both the initial cause of cell injury and the consequences of such injury. In trauma, inflammation is triggered by pathogens, tissue necrosis, and foreign bodies. The inflammatory cascade is amplified by early recruitment of inflammatory cells, which in turn release further mediators. In the setting of trauma, the amount of inflammation is usually determined by the amount of energy transferred to the soft tissue and bone, the degree of contamination, and type of bacteria, if any, present, as well as patient factors, such as preexisting immunodeficiency, diabetes, or steroid use. The magnitude of the inflammatory response depends on the severity of the injury and the degree of vascularization of the tissue that is injured. Inflammation is likely initiated by cellular damage and subsequent leakage of intracellular contents, as well as by capillary damage, leading to blood flow into the site of injury and initiation of the injury hematoma.

Inflammation is primarily represented by four major events: vasodilatation, increased micro vascular permeability, cellular activation and adhesion of immune cells, and coagulation. Vasodilatation and increased permeability of microvasculature permit extravasations of protein-rich fluid into tissues. This fluid consists of macrophages and monocytes, which release and stimulate cytokines and growth factors. Loss of fluid and increased vessel diameter lead to slower blood flow and vascular congestion. Once leukocytes have been recruited to the site of injury, they are activated by intracellular components in the extracellular space, by proteins expressed on the surface of dead cells, or by cytokines.

Inflammatory Mediators

There are several important mediators in inflammation. They can be categorized into cell-derived mediators, which may be sequestered into granules (histamine) or synthesized de novo (prostaglandins, cytokines), and plasma-derived mediators, which circulate as inactive precursors. Active mediators are produced in response to substances released from necrotic cells or microbes, and one mediator can stimulate the release of others. Platelets are an important source of cytokines and growth factors, and they are stimulated to release these cellular products during clotting, which occurs when platelets come in contact with collagen immediately after trauma is sustained. There is increasing interest in the orthopedic community on the use of platelet enriched products as a therapeutic option for a variety of musculoskeletal conditions, ranging from tendon injury to bony nonunions. Histamine is present in mast cell granules and can be released in response to trauma, producing dilatation of arterioles and increased permeability of venules. Prostaglandins are a group cell derived mediators that can cause vasodilation, fever, and pain. The mechanism of NSAIDs' (non steroidal anti-inflammatory) anti-inflammatory action is by inhibiting cyclooxygenase, which is an enzyme that is critical in prostaglandin formation. Leukotrienes increase vascular permeability and cause chemotaxis and leukocyte adhesion.

Cytokines exert their effects by binding to specific cellular receptors and are thus able to regulate gene transcription and modify intracellular signally pathways, both locally and systemically. They have small molecular weight and are active in extremely low concentrations. They have overlapping functions, multiple targets, and pleiotrophic actions. TNFa and IL-1 are two important early pro-inflammatory cytokines. They affect a wide variety of cells to induce fever, production of cytokines, endothelial gene regulation, chemotaxis, leukocyte adherence, and activation of fibroblasts. They are responsible for the systemic effects of inflammation, such as loss of appetite and tachycardia. IL-6 is another cytokine that appears to be critical in the inflammatory cascade in the setting of trauma. IL-6 levels are elevated 60 minutes after trauma (or surgery) and decline over days 2 to 5 after trauma. Importantly, the magnitude of IL-6 elevation after mechanical trauma can be used as a reliable marker for the magnitude of systemic inflammation and correlates with the risk of post-injury complications. IL-6 appears to be responsible for regulating the acute phase response.

Systemic Response

The inflammatory cytokines act locally, as well as systemically, and can lead to signs and symptoms similar to sepsis, including hypotension, fever, fatigue, anorexia, headache, activation of coagulation, and other systemic changes known together as the Systemic Inflammatory Response Syndrome (SIRS). This syndrome is most commonly seen in the setting of a serious bacterial infection and is initiated by circulating bacteria triggering an intense systemic inflammatory response. SIRS however does not require a setting of infection and can occur only as the result of injury and an inflammatory cascade. There is recent evidence that the systemic release of mitochondrial DNA and mitochondrial molecular patterns, which can occur with cellular breakdown in trauma, play a role in activating systemic inflammation in SIRS that is not a result of bacterial infection. Mitochondrial DNA and molecular patterns are similar to that of bacteria because they were likely derived from similar ancestors prior to the incorporation of mitochondria into human cells. Because of this similarity mitochondrial DNA and molecular patterns may trigger this intense inflammatory response by binding to the same immune receptors that recognize circulating bacteria.

SIRS can be of severe consequence to the already debilitated trauma patient, resulting in pulmonary function collapse and organ failure. Careful consideration of timing is critical in the care of the trauma patients since further surgical intervention can worsen the inflammatory response. In severe polytrauma patients, it is often preferable to perform limited fracture stabilization, rather than definitive orthopaedic repair immediately, since surgery can function as a second traumatic event with a second wave of inflammatory cytokine release, which can augment the initial systemic inflammatory response to the trauma with increased potential to cause systemic disease including SIRS and ARDS (Second hit theory). SIRS is universal after traumatic injury and that the clinical presentation differs only in intensity. One study showed that combined fracture and soft tissue injury caused higher levels of systemic inflammatory mediators (IL-6 and IL-10) than either fracture of soft tissue injury alone. The femoral fracture being the primary model since it is a long bone fracture and is often most related with systemic and pulmonary collapse secondary to injury and surgery. Concern about the timing of definitive intramedullary fixation, which includes intramedullary reaming and further release of marrow contents and inflammatory mediators, is an ongoing debate in the orthopedic trauma community. It has been clear for several decades that early surgical stabilization of long-bone fractures reduces pulmonary complications when compared to limb placed in a splint or skeletal traction. However, patients who are hemodynamically unstable, hypothermic, who have coagulation abnormalities or poor oxygenation due to traumatic lung injury have increased rates of acute lung injury after intermedullary reaming. If these conditions cannot be reversed with adequate resuscitation, these patients benefit from a protocol of damage control orthopaedics consisting of initial external fixation for transient stabilization followed by delayed definitive fracture fixation stabilization followed by delayed definitive fracture fixation.

Although inflammation is potentially harmful, with the ability to induce both local and systemic responses, it is also necessary to initiate the healing process. The inflammatory cells and proteins release growth factors and chemokines that recruit stem cells and other precursors and immune cells to the site of injury. These are then activated and stimulate others into becoming mitogenically active and proliferative. Even the hematoma and fibrin clot that occurs at the time of injury is important, likely providing a provisional structure for regenerative cells. Studies demonstrate that when inflammation is limited, either in knockout mice or by pharmacological intervention, healing does not occur normally or is disrupted in time and sequence.

Bone Material and Structural Properties

Because the human musculoskeletal system is a living organ with predominantly a mechanical role, both physiology and engineering principles are critical for its study and understanding. The critical feature of any structural design is to consider what loads the structure must sustain and to adjust the overall geometry and the materials used to achieve the desired function. This is true in the musculoskeletal system as well.

The main function of the musculoskeletal system is to support and protect soft tissues and to assist with movement. Bones, muscle, tendons, ligaments and joints function to generate and to transfer forces so that our limbs can be manipulated in three-dimensional space. The musculoskeletal system also has a metabolic role in calcium handling, as well as hematopoiesis. To optimize function, bones must be rigid enough that they don't fail when loaded or demonstrate unnatural elastic behavior. They must also be elastic enough to absorb energy when loaded, but not so elastic that they are subject to plastic deformation. The primary function of the musculoskeletal system is to manage applied load. The ability of a bone to resist fracture depends on the intrinsic properties of the material and the spatial distribution of bone mass (geometry and micro architecture).

Material Properties

Material properties characterize the behavior of materials comprising the tissue and to a first approximation, are independent of the size of the tissue. They are usually expressed in terms of the stress-strain relationship of the material. Stress is the amount of force applied per unit area, and strain represents the degree of deformation in response to a specific stress. Elastic deformation is the component of the stress-strain relationship in which the material deforms as load is applied yet returns to its original shape when the load is removed. The slope of this curve is the elastic modulus or Young's modulus and it is a measure of stiffness. The stiffer the material is, the steeper the slope (the less it deforms under stress). Bone is an anisotropic material with a nonlinear stress-strain relationship that can be approximated as linear in its elastic region. When bone is loaded in the elastic range it absorbs the energy by shortening and widening in compression, lengthening and narrowing in tension, and then returning to its original length when unloaded. Plastic deformation describes the condition in which some permanent deformation remains after the load is removed. With regards to bone, deformation in the plastic zone includes micro-cracks and disruption of collagen fibrils and its trabecular architecture. The anelastic modulus describes the slope of the stress-strain curve in the plastic range. Once the load exceeds the plastic deformation zone, the energy is dissipated in fracture or tissue failure. The yield point is the point at which elastic behavior changes to plastic, and it essentially describes the safe functional load. Subtle changes in density, which can occur with aging, disease, use and disuse, greatly change strength and elastic modulus.

Material properties of bone are generally separated into the material properties of the outer cortex and material properties of trabecular bone, which is found inside the cortex.

These structures serve slightly different purposes and this is reflected by their material properties as well as the architecture. Bone is an anisotropic material; the stress-strain behavior differs with different directions of loading. Cortical bone is stronger and stiffer when loaded in the longitudinal direction than in the transverse direction. This is related to the orientation of bone microstructure. The orientation of orbicular architecture corresponds with the orientation of the principle stress sustained by the tissue. In less anisotropic bone, trabecular bone consists of cylindrical struts extending about 1mm before making connection with other struts, usually at right angles. In more highly anisotropic bone, trabeculi are more sheet-like than cylindrical, and they are longer and preferentially aligned in one direction. On a molecular scale, regions of bone loaded in tension tend to have their collagen fibers oriented longitudinally, while those loaded in compression tend to be oriented obliquely to transversely and collagen fibrils have been found to be oriented in the direction of the trabeculae. Because of the anisotropic nature of bone, there is not a single value for elastic modulus and hardness of cortical or trabecular bone. This anisotropic nature will play an important role in bone resistance to failure or fracture.

Bone mineral content contributes to stiffness of bone at the expense of flexibility, and it also has an effect on bone toughness. As mineral content increases up to 65%, toughness increases, and as mineral content exceeds about 65%, toughness begins to decline. Toughness is determined by the material composition and the ability of the microstructure to dissipate deformation energy without propagation of a crack. Energy can be dissipated by viscoelastic flow and by the formation of non-connected micro-cracks. Collagen cross-links are known to limit crack propagation, thus increasing bone toughness. Collagen structure is another important contributor to bone material properties. The triple helix of collagen and its cross-links confer strength in tension and are closely related to post-yield properties of bone, particularly bone toughness and ductility. Water content also plays a role in relative stiffness and toughness of bone. The collagen network is very sensitive to the condition of hydration. Dehydrated bone exhibits increased stiffness and decreased toughness. The literature on documenting the mechanical properties of bone in various forms of loading is extensive.

Bone also exhibits viscoelastic behavior; bone strength depends on rate of loading and it exhibits creep and stress-relaxation. At higher strain rates, both ultimate strength and elastic modulus increase. Under constant loads, bone will continue to deform or creep. If the strain is held constant, the stress decreases with time (relaxation). If cyclic loading is applied hysteresis (a phase lag in which the shape of the unloading curve is different from the shape of the loading curve), occurs leading to a dissipation of mechanical energy. More simply, some solid materials can flow slightly, but not indefinitely, and the rate of flow is proportional to the load being imposed but also inversely proportional to some function of time that the load has been imposed.

Bone also exhibits fatigue, in which loads below the yield point applied in succession progressively create a crack that grows until the material fails at a stress that is below the yield point. The fatigue resistance of a material depends more on limiting micro-crack growth than micro-crack initiation, and in bone, fatigue resistance also depends how quickly the material is able to restore micro-cracks, or heal. Micro-crack propagation is limited by bone heterogeneity and microstructural features, like cement lines around each osteon and the interface between loose and dense lamellae. However, unlike inert materials, bone is able to sense accumulation of micro damage and to repair it. The phenomenon of fatigue is responsible for stress fractures, which are commonly seen in athletes, like runners, who do not provide frequently loaded bones with the opportunity to repair micro-damage.

Structural Properties

Structural properties of the musculoskeletal system, which characterize the tissue in its intact form, also play a critical role in managing applied loads and particularly in transferring stress through the skeletal system. This takes into account the material properties of each type of tissue in the structure, as well as the geometry and architecture of the system. Overall strength of the system depends on the size and shape of the bone (cortical thickness, cross sectional area and moment of inertia), the micro-architecture of the bone (cortical porosity, trabecular morphology), and the amount of accumulated damage.

Moment of inertia is a measure of how the material is distributed in the cross-section of the object relative to the load applied to it, and moment of inertia can be used to predict the resistance of the structure to bending and deflection.

$$\text{Moment of inertia} = P(R^4 - r^4)/4$$

R = cortical outer diameter; r = cortical inner diameter

Since moment of inertia is proportional to the diameter of the structure to the 4th power small increases in external diameter of a long bone can markedly improve its resistance to bending and torsional loading. Resistance to compressive loading depends on the cross sectional area of bone; resistance to bending and torsional loads involves distributing bone material far from the neutral axis of bending or torsion (generally this axis is near the center of bone). This is highly relevant for understating changes in bone properties with aging. Osteoporosis as a result of aging, not only results in decreased mineral bone content, but aging causes a architectural remodeling which affects the moment of inertia of bone. Geriatric patients have long bones characterized by an increase in external diameter and a larger increase in internal diameter, resulting in a thinner cortex. The increased inner diameter (and thinner cortex) results in significant decreases in bone bending resistance since moment of inertia is directly related to $(R^4 - r^4)$. This is countered, to some degree by the increase in outer cortical diameter.

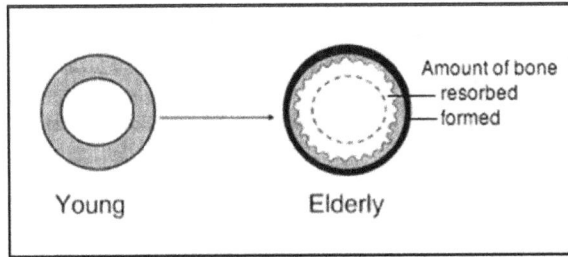

Change in bone cortical diameter with age.

Geometry is difficult to discuss in general over the entire skeleton because it is not uniform; skeletal structure and geometry is specific to the needs of each anatomical region. For example, long bones are needed for loading and movement, and rigidity in these bones is therefore favored over flexibility. By shifting the cortical shell outward from the neutral axis, the long bones have increased bending strength. External and internal contours differ at each point along and around the shaft, reflecting local modeling and remodeling in response to regional loading needs. The reverse is true in the vertebrae, where ability to deform in response to loading is favored over stiffness. Vertebral bodies with large volume of trabecular bone function more like springs than levers. Interconnecting trabecular plates achieve lightness and favor structural flexibility over stiffness. Additionally the diameter and thickness of bones is different, depending on the types of stresses that are sustained by that bone. For example, the femoral neck adjacent to the shaft is elliptical, with the longer diameter in the superior-inferior direction with greater cortical thickness inferiorly. These geometrical features minimize bending. Near the femoral head, stresses are mainly compressive and the geometry reflects this. The femoral neck is more circular and largely trabecular, with a cortex of similar thickness around its perimeter.

Remodeling

In 1982, Julius Wolff published a paper on bone remodeling, defining a phenomenon that would become known as Wolff's law--that bone changes external geometry and internal architecture in response to stresses acting on it. Wolff's law has been quoted in numerous ways through the years and referenced for support whenever the argument of stress modulated bone remodeling was being made. However, Wolf's law is not a law in the quantitative sense but rather an insightful observation. There is no known growth law for bone or any other musculoskeletal tissue that is universally applicable or demonstrated. It is also unclear if bone remodeling is a stress- or strain-governed phenomenon.

During the remodeling process, osteoclasts (bone resorption cells) remove old bone tissue by resorption, and osteoblasts (bone forming cells) create new bone tissue. It is understood that bone is remodeled to meet its mechanical demands. There is evidence that micro damage initiates bone remodeling and that fracture repair is a form of load-induced bone remodeling in which damage serves as trigger. Stress fractures are often localized radiographically when patients complain of limb pain, and a radiograph demonstrates a reactive response or fracture callus that illustrates the remodeling process initiated by the injury. The principles of remodeling and bone fracture healing with callus often reflect the need to redistribute stress at the site of healing. A large callus that increases the cross sectional areal of the bone at the site of a transverse shaft fracture serves a means of increasing the moment of inertia and decreasing the bending stress sustained at the fracture site.

Evidence for exercise-induced osseous remodeling in adults is less clear. Data from intervention randomized control trials is limited. Follow-up times have been short, the quality of the conduction of intervention and reporting of outcomes has been poor, and there has been a lack of reporting on the specific exercise characteristics that are effective. However, adaptation to loading in children and adolescents is well documented, and these changes in bone density and geometry persist into adulthood. Exercise, particularly weight-bearing impact exercises, in prepubertal boys increases estimates of bone strength at loaded sites, likely due to thicker cortices. Young tennis players have increased cortical thickness and increased cortical drift in the perosteal direction in their playing arm compared with their non-dominant arm. However, in middle-aged subjects, tennis did not stimulate cortical drift in the periosteal direction. In middle-aged subjects cross-sectional areas of the radius were actually smaller, suggesting that unilateral use of the arm after the third decade of life suppresses age-related changes in bone geometry since normally there is increased endocortical area and slower expansion of periosteal area resulting in decreased cortical thickness. There is some evidence that exercise can increase bone mineral density (BMD) in post-menopausal women, particularly after one year or longer. The type of exercise and the amount of improvement is somewhat contested. A few studies, however, suggest that resistance training and low- to moderate-impact exercises are most effective. However the gains in BMD are generally small (1-2%). Exercise has been shown to result in up to a 50% reduction in fracture incidence, but a large component of this reduction is likely due to improved muscle function and balance, combined with the small 1-2% increase in BMD.

The cellular mechanism for remodeling control is a focus of research interest, but the details are still largely unknown. Osteocytes appear to be the primary mechanosensors that begin the remodeling cascade. There is evidence that pressure gradients within the bone matrix lead to interstitial fluid flow in the lacunar-canalicular system, which activates mechanosensory osteocytes that reside in lacunae. The osteocytes then transmit load-provoked signals via canaliculi and gap junctions. There is evidence that osteocyte death is associated with remodeling as well. Death of cells likely creates biochemical and chemotactic signals, which indicate presence of damage and its location. Regions of micro damage contain apoptotic osteocytes whereas quiescent zones do not.

Mechanics of Bone Regeneration

Under most circumstances bone is able to regenerate its baseline mechanical properties after sustaining a fracture. However, the mechanical environment is critical in establishing tissue formation patterns during fracture repair. There are two forms of bone healing: direct or primary healing and indirect or secondary healing, which occur depending on the mechanical environment. Direct healing occurs when the fracture is subjected to surgical fixation with absolute stability, fixation with absolute stability, with no interfragmentary motion or strain with no interfragmentary motion or strain. This direct healing is achieved by interfragmentary compression, most often achieved technically during surgery with lag screws and/or compression plates. In this setting, bone heals via intramembranous ossification without development of a fracture callus. This is most often applied to peri-articular fractures where perfect anatomic reduction is necessary for an optimal functional outcome. Indirect healing occurs when the fracture is subjected to relative stability, or when there is some degree of interfragmentary motion or strain. Bone heals with development of a fracture callus, which changes the mechanical properties and the geometry of the fracture site. This often produces optimal biological conditions for healing.

Interfragmentary strain theory, is the basis for our understanding of how the mechanical environment impacts tissue differentiation in a fracture gap. He theorized that the magnitude of interfragmentary strain determines subsequent tissue differentiation of fracture gap tissue. Each tissue has different strain tolerances, and applied interfragmentary strain must be smaller than the strain tolerance of a tissue for it to form. Strains below 2% permit direct bone formation (direct fracture healing), strains below 10% allow cartilage differentiation and subsequent endocondral ossification (indirect fracture healing), and strains between 10% and 100% lead to granulation tissue formation and non-union. Perren believed that differentiation of initial fracture gap tissue would stiffen the fracture gap leading to lower interfragmentary strain, allowing differentiation to the next stiffest tissue.

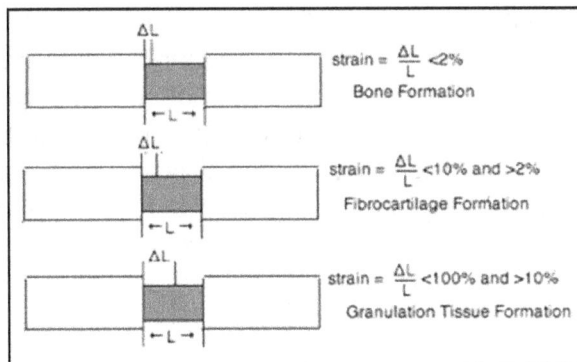

Interfragmentary strain theory. The formation of tissue type based on strain at the fracture gap.

In addition to strain magnitude, both the type of mechanical stimulus (cyclic, compressive, tensile or shear) and the degree of vascular supply would affect tissue differentiation. A different mechanoregulation concept proposed two biophysical stimuli, shear strain in the solid phase and fluid velocity in the interstitial fluid phase. According to this concept, bone formed only when both stimuli were low enough. However, none of these models are flawless, and clinical results suggest that these theories are correct in the extremes, where they are similar: low strain leads to bone formation, and high strain leads to fibrous non-union.

Geriatric Biomechanics

Osteoporosis

Osteoporosis is defined as a "systemic skeletal disease characterized by low bone mass and micro-architectural deterioration of bone tissue, leading to enhanced bone fragility and a consequent increase in fracture risk. In the US over 1.5 million fractures occur each year, including 280,000 hip fractures, and these numbers are expected to double or triple in the coming decades due to the aging population. There are several components of whole bone strength that change over time, including the intrinsic properties of the materials that form bone, the amount of bone (i.e. mass), and the spatial distribution of bone mass (ie geometry and microarchitecture). The biggest challenge is determining the effects of these changes and identifying which change is most important in the development of osteoprosis.

Bone Mechanical Properties

Whole bone strength declines dramatically with age. Changes that occur in cortical, as well as trabecular bone collectively lead to decreased bone strength and increased risk of fracture. Between 30 and 80 years of age, elastic modulus of cortical bone decreases by 8%, bone strength decreases by 11%, and toughness declines by 34%. All of these changes result in mechanical failure or fracture as a result of lower energy traumatic events. The specific changes that contribute to these events are a topic of investigation. It is clear that there is a reduction in overall bone mass with age. It is thought that thinning of cortical bone and increased porosity are major contributors to loss in stiffness, strength, toughness, and resistance to propagation of cracks. Studies have shown that there is a four-fold increase in cortical bone porosity from 20 to 80 years of age. The elastic modulus of cortical bone in a longitudinal direction decreases significantly with increased porosity. Other factors that may contribute to decreased toughness include loss of bone mass, increased mineralization or development of hypermineralized regions, accumulation of micro damage, decreased integrity of collagen, and changes in collagen crosslinks.

The changes in mechanical properties of trabecular bone are even more pronounced. Between 30 and 80 years of age, elastic modulus of trabecular bone decreases by 64%, strength decreases by 68%, and toughness decreases by 70%. These changes are likely due to loss of trabecaular plates and connectivity, as well as micro damage. Studies have shown that loss of connectivity in trabecular plates produces a greater deficit in bone strength than thinned plates that continue to be well connected.

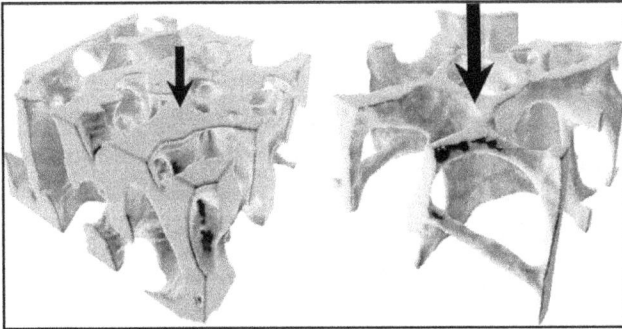

Loss of trabecular bone mass and decreased trabecular connectivity ocurs with increasing age.

Bone Geometry

The overall size and shape of bones play important roles in their mechanical behavior. Microarchitectural changes in trabecular bone, such as decreased number of trabecular plates and decreased connectivity between plates, appear to play a large role in decreased strength of trabecular bone. Decreases in bone mass and changes in distribution of bone mass also appear to play a large role in overall bone strength. It is well established that endosteal expansion (increase in inner cortical radius due to loss of cortical bone) and perioesteal expansion (increase in external cortical radius due to deposition of new bone on the external surface of bone cortex) both occur, but that endosteal expansion exceeds periosteal expansion. This excess leads to age-related deceases in cortical thickness but increases in bone outer diameter. Decreased cortical thickness contributes to the decreases in strength, elastic modulus, and toughness of bone. However, the greater diameter increases moment of inertia and increases structural resistance to bending and torsional loads, which may offset decreases in cortical thickness and bone mineral density that occur with age. This effect explains how bone mineral density can decrease while bending resistance may not.

Bone is known to be highly anisotropic at baseline and is strongest in the direction of habitual loading. There is emerging evidence to suggest that in hip-fracture patients, bone is more anisotropic and more highly oriented in the direction of habitual loading than control subjects, occurring at the expense of strength in other directions. One study examined specimens from hip fracture patients and un-fractured controls, and controlled for bone volume. The study found that hip fracture specimens of the same bone volume were more highly organized in the direction of habitual loading. This increased anisotropy leads to a reduced ability to withstand off-axis impact, during a fall in a direction different from the direction of habitual loading, such as a sideways fall. In these patients, bone reorganization may be overcompensating for the low mass status by increasing the degree of anisotropy so that strength of the bone is only maximized in the frequently loaded direction.

The rate of bone remodeling may also play a role in development of osteoporosis. During growth the balance between bone that is removed and bone that is formed is positive (more bone is added than removed). Once skeletal maturity is reached, this reverses and the balance becomes negative (more bone is removed than is added in the remodeling process). In general, the rate of remodeling, and therefore the rate of bone loss, is extremely slow later in life. However, there is evidence to suggest that estrogen deficiency increases the rate of remodeling and there may be other factors that modulate remodeling rate. It is possible that bone loss is driven more by increased rate of remodeling than by magnitude of bone loss during each remodeling event. Another possible mechanism through which bone remodeling contributes to osteoporosis is through increasing dysfunction of mechanoreceptors, which drive the remodeling process. This could contribute to bone loss and could interfere with remodeling in response to micro damage or in response to changes in loading.

Bone Mineral Density

Bone mineral density (BMD) is the attribute currently used in clinical practice to diagnose osteoporosis and to monitor efficacy of interventions. Dual-emission X-ray absorptiometry (DXA) is used to measure BMD clinically. BMD is bone mineral content (BMC) (measured as the attenuation of the X-ray by the bones being scanned) divided by area of the site being scanned. Osteoporosis is diagnosed by determining how many standard deviations the BMD of the patient is below the mean BMD of a healthy thirty year-old. Any BMD that is greater than two and a half standard deviations below the mean thirty year-old BMD is considered osteoporotic.

BMD explains a significant portion of the risk of osteoporotic fracture and correlates with bone strength. BMD is a strong predictor of fracture risk; risk of fracture increases 50-150% with each standard deviation decrease in bone mass as measured by DXA. However, it is clear that there are other factors that contribute to fracture risk. Studies have demonstrated that there is a significant overlap in BMD between osteoporotic individuals and healthy individuals who have not experienced osteoporotic fracture. The risk of fracture of the hip or forearm in a 75 year-old is 4-7 times that of a 45 year-old with an identical BMD. Risk for hip fracture actually doubles for each decade of age increase even after adjusting for bone density. Additionally, current therapies are able to, at best, increase bone density by 10%, but the risk of fracture decreases by a much larger extent. The specific non-BMD factors that explain this discrepancy are not known.

BMD is used clinically because it represents a non-invasive, relatively inexpensive way, to predict fracture risk. It indirectly reflects bone geometry, mass, size, and mineralization. However, DXA does not provide information on cortical vs. cancellous density, 3D geometry, trabecular architecture, microstructure or strength parameters. It functions as a surrogate for these attributes, which are difficult to measure non-invasively.

Bisphosphonates

Bisphosphonates are a class of drugs that are commonly used to manage osteoporosis. They function by inhibiting bone resorption by osteoclasts, which occurs during remodeling. They mimic the structure of pyrophosphate and are incorporated into bone. They are then ingested by osteoclasts and ultimately result in osteoclast cell death. During bisphosphonate treatment bone remodeling rate is slower and there are a fewer number of osteoclast-induced excavation sites each with decreased depth, leading to slower bone loss. Fractures are less frequent but not eliminated in patients taking bisphosphonates. Maximum fracture risk reduction occurs in the first year of treatment. Observed fracture risk appears to be at least twice as large as would be expected from changes in BMD alone.

In recent years, there has been some controversy with regard to safety of prolonged bisphosphonate administration. Several case series initially described cases of "atypical" subtrochanteric and diaphyseal femur fractures and suggested that the risk may be increased in long-term users of bisphosphonates. Unique clinical features of these fractures in the literature include prodromal pain for weeks to months prior to fracture, complete absence of precipitating trauma, and bilateral fracture (either simultaneous or sequential) in some. Distinctive radiographic features include presence of a stress reaction on the affected and/or unaffected side, transverse or short oblique pattern (in contrast to the more common spiral fracture), thick femoral cortices, and unicortical breaking. The theory behind this concern is that long-term bisphosphonate use with prolonged suppression of bone turnover may lead to accumulation of micro damage due to impaired remodeling. It has also been suggested that long-term bisphosphonate use could create a more homogenous tissue with BMD more similar throughout, and this may offer less resistance to propagation of cracking. Fracture patterns and cortical thickening are reminiscent of osteopetrosis and fractures that occur in ostepetrosis in the subtrochanteric area. Osteopetrosis is a congenital malfunction of the osteoclast resulting in severe brittle and dense bone. There are several retrospective cohort studies that indicate that there is a correlation between atypical subtrochanteric and diaphyseal femur fractures and use of several bisphosphonates. However, it is difficult to determine whether this correlation is confounded by the fact that those taking bisphosphonates, particularly long-term, have significant osteoporosis that may account for these atypical fractures. Data from three large placebo controlled, randomized control trials have indicated that there is no association between bisphosphonate use and atypical subtrochanteric or diaphyseal femur fracture. Based on these three studies, it is likely that these subtrochanteric and femoral shaft fractures may be related to the underlying osteoporosis, which was the reason for long-term bisphosphonate use or to an additional metabolic predisposition yet to be diagnosed. However, confidence intervals in these studies were high due to the small number of events, and, although, one study followed patients for ten years, it is possible that this is not long enough to observe an effect. Additionally, it has been suggested that these fractures are associated with bisphosphonate use in a subset of patients, like those taking steroids or proton pump inhibitors.

Fracture Mechanisms

Injury patterns sustained in trauma can often be inferred from bone radiographs after trauma with certain confidence and consistency. Knowledge of patterns of injury attributed to specific modes of trauma can be used to predict associated injuries, since not all injuries are obvious at presentation. This knowledge also serves to develop or to improve safety features and equipment.

The magnitude, type and direction of forces, as well as material properties of bone and surrounding structures, dictate the fracture pattern to a certain degree. Severity of injury is determined by peak forces and moments resulting from the impact and the tissues' resistance to injury. The greater the energy absorbed by the bone, the more severe the fracture and the more likely that comminution and displacement will occur. Tissues surrounding bone, including muscle, tendons, ligaments, fat and skin, can affect fracture pattern by absorbing some of the load energy and also by creating additional load. The main factors that affect the load at which bone fails include bone geometry, bone material properties, load application point, load direction and the rate of load application. The main load bearing structure in bone is the cortex, which is denser, has greater volume and mass, and is in a location that makes it more capable of sustaining large loads. Trabecular bone largely functions to direct stresses to cortical bone. Multiple injuries can be caused by the same mechanism because forces can be transmitted along the entire length of a bone or through several bones, causing damage anywhere along the way.

Simple Fracture Patterns

There are a limited number of loading modes that bone can be subjected to, and these result in predictable fracture patterns. Complex fracture patterns occur when multiple loading modes and directions are applied during the same event. Loading modes include tensile loading, compressive loading, shear loading, bending load, and loading in torsion. Bone is weakest in tension and strongest in compression. When bone is loaded in tension it tends to fracture along a transverse plane that is approximately perpendicular to the direction of loading. When undergoing a compressive load, bone will fail secondary to shear stress since shear strength of bone is much less than compressive strength. During compressive loading, shear stresses develop at a plane that is approximately 45 degrees from the long axis of the bone, and it is along this oblique plan that bone fails. Max shear stress is approximately one half of the applied compressive stress. Bending is essentially a combination of tensile and compressive loading. When bone is undergoing bending, high tensile stresses develop on the convex side and high compressive stresses develop on the concave side. A transverse fracture is initiated on the tensile side, and two oblique fractures occur on the compressive side, creating what is referred to as a butterfly fragment. Fracture secondary to torsion usually begins at a small defect at the bone surface, and then the fracture follows a spiral pattern along planes of high tensile stress, since bone is weakest in tension. It is a worthwhile exercise for a traumatologist to carefully look at a radiograph after trauma and to recreate the mechanism of fracture based on the fracture pattern. More complex and comminuted fracture patterns are essentially a combination of these simple patterns. Materials properties of bone can be approximated as isotropic when load is delivered at a high rate.

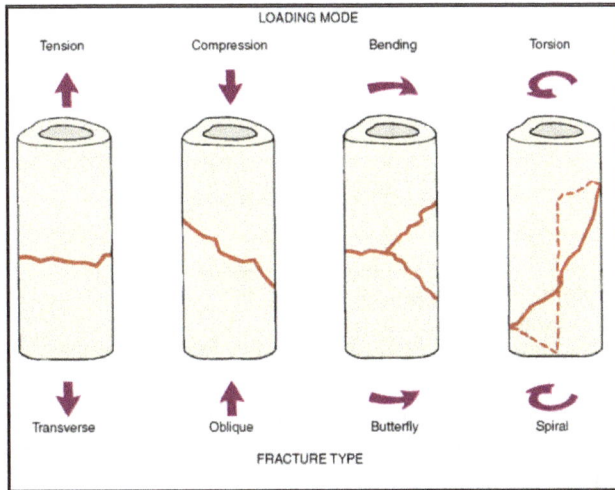

Simple fracture patterns which occur as a result of loading mode.

Fall

Fall is an important source of musculoskeletal injury and accounts for 87% of fracture in older adults. The two most common injuries secondary to fall are hip fractures and upper extremity fractures, and in some instances, they are related in that impacts at the wrist have been shown to modulate or lessen impacts at the pelvis during lateral and forward falls. This requires rapid reaction and movement times, as well as arm muscle strength, all of which decrease with age to some degree. One study measured reaction time of young and elderly women and found that the typical elderly female is able move her hands quickly enough to break a forward fall, but not a sideways fall, while young women are able to break both types of fall.

Fall on Outstretched Hand

Fall on outstretched hand is a classic mechanism of injury leading to fracture of the scaphoid bone of the hand, fracture of the distal ulna and radius, fracture-dislocation of the elbow, fracture dislocation of the shoulder and fracture of the clavicle. This injury mechanism accounts for approximately 90% of fractures at the distal radius, humeral neck, and supracondylar elbow region. During a fall on a stiff surface, hand contact force occurs in two stages: the first is a high-frequency peak load which corresponds to a large deceleration of arm mass, which occurs at the wrist at the moment of impact; the second is a low-frequency oscillation with a lower peak force, which is due to deformation of the shoulder spring. Increases in body mass more strongly increase the peak magnitude of the low-frequency component, and increases in fall height more dramatically increase the high-frequency component.

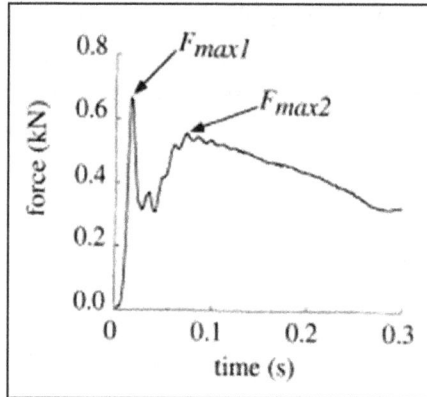

Impact response of the body during a forward fall onto the outstretched hand. Measures of hand contact force during this event show a high-frequency transient (with associated peak force Fmax1) followed by a lower-frequency oscillation (with associated peak force Fmax2).

The fracture pattern depends on the force magnitude, on how force is distributed across the bones of the hand, and on how it is transmitted to other upper extremity structures. The magnitude and distribution of contact force during a fall also depends on the configuration of the body at impact and on the soft tissue thickness over the palm region. The weakest area on the palm is over the scaphoid and lunate, which articulate directly with and transmit force to the distal radius. A fall with peak force localized to this area is most likely to result in fracture.

Understanding the mechanics of an injury helps to develop preventative measures. In one study patients were able to learn to reduce the impact force applied to the distal forearm by 27% by slightly flexing their elbows and reducing the velocity of the hands relative to the torso. Another study showed that a 5mm foam pad reduced peak pressure and peak force by 83% and 13% respectively, which can represent the difference between a fracture and isolated soft tissue damage. Additionally weight plays a role in degree of loading during a fall. Peak pressure was 77% higher in individuals with high body mass index (BMI) when compared to low BMI participants. In contrast to what we see in the hip, having high BMI is not associated with increased thickness of soft tissue in the hand, and therefore the extra body mass contributed to the total force of the fall without providing extra tissue to absorb the energy.

Femoral Neck Fracture

Hip fracture or femoral neck fracture is a significant source of morbidity in the elderly population, and 90% of such fractures are due to fall from standing. Hip fracture in the elderly is associated with a 20% chance of death and a 25% risk of long-term institutionalization. Changes that occur with aging in the material properties of bone play a significant role in femoral neck fracture; however, the mechanics of the fall (direction, location of impact) are critical as well. Although 90% of hip fractures are due to a fall, only 1% of falls actually result in hip fracture, which is surprising from a biomechanical perspective because the energy available during a fall from standing often exceeds that required to fracture both elderly and young proximal femurs. Mitigating factors can be many.

The femoral neck undergoes constant bending loads during normal weight-bearing activities. Compressive force through the femoral head can range from 4-8 times the body weight during normal activities and this force acts through a significant moment arm (the length of the femoral neck), which causes large bending loads on the femoral neck. In normal gait the greatest stresses occur in the subcapital and mid-femoral neck regions. Within these regions maximum compressive stresses occur inferiorly where the cortex is thick and smaller tensile stresses occur superiorly where the cortex is thinner. Sideways falls with impact to the greater trochanter are the events most directly related to hip fracture in older adults. The femoral neck is weakest when the posterolateral aspect of the greater trochanter is impacted. During a sideways fall on the greater trochanter, the stress state is reversed from normal ambulation and the greatest compressive stresses occur in the superior femoral neck while the smaller tensile stresses occur in the inferior region. The superior cortex of the femoral neck is significantly thinner in older than younger individuals, while the inferior cortex is significantly thicker in older than younger individuals. Therefore, during a sideways fall, which is more frequent in the elderly, the large compressive stress occurs in the superior cortex, which is thinner and more likely to fail in the elderly. Multiple studies have suggested that proximal femur fractures are typically initiated by a failure in the superior aspect of the femoral neck, followed by a failure in the inferior aspect of the femoral neck. Subjects with a longer moment arm in the context of a sideways fall increases the force applied to the hip and predisposes the subject to a hip fracture. Hip axis length and neck-shaft angle both contribute to the moment arm of the hip and both have been independently shown to predict hip fracture. A fall onto the greater trochanter may also generate an axial force along the femoral neck, resulting in an impaction fracture. Additionally, investigators have reported that the lower extremity externally rotates during a fall and that, at the extremes of external rotation, the femoral neck impinges against the posterior acetabular rim. The acetabular rim then acts like a fulcrum to concentrate the stress experienced by that region at time of impact.

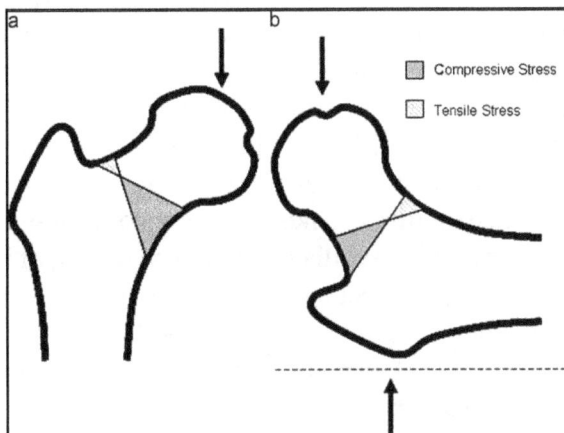

The magnitude and nature of the stresses on the femoral neck differ depending on the applied load. For example in (a) walking: the inferior surface tends to be subjected to a large component of compressive stress, while the superior surface is subjected to a smaller tensile stress and (b) sideways fall on the greater trochanter: the inferior surface tends to be subjected to a small tensile stress, while the superior surface is subjected to a larger compressive stress.

Since only a small fraction of falls actually result in fracture and the energy available in a fall is sufficient to fracture the proximal femur, there are mitigating factors that affect the actual impact forces. Some of these include soft tissue properties and body positioning at the time of impact. Energy of a fall can be dissipated by contracting muscles; this contraction is likely done more effectively in younger patients than older patients with slower, weaker muscles. Substantial energy can also be absorbed by skin and fat overlying the hip region. Peak femoral impact force actually decreases in a linear manner with increasing soft-tissue thickness at a rate of approximately 79 N per 1mm change in thickness, and peak pressure over the greater trochanter averaged 266% higher in low BMI participants than in high BMI participants in another study. Additionally, there are actions that fallers can take to moderate the force applied directly to the femur. Falling techniques can be taught to geriatric patients by physical therapists. In one study young subjects were able to impact the outstretched hand and pelvis near-simultaneously during an unexpected fall which distributed the body's impact energy. Fallers can also produce "energy absorbing" work during descent, which occurs by eccentrically contracting lower extremity muscles, which increases the vertical component of foot reaction forces resulting in decreased downward acceleration. Mats as thin as 1.5cm have been shown to decrease peak hip impact force by 8% and thicker mats have a greater effect. Ultimately, these modifiable factors, which diminish the peak impact force, are critical because they represent ways that hip fracture can be reduced or prevented.

Motor Vehicle Collision

Motor vehicle collision is a common source of polytrauma, injuring more than 5 million people every year. Generally, injuries are sustained when the vehicle rapidly decelerates while the vehicle occupant continues to move at previous speeds. When the body absorbs energy beyond its tolerance fracture or injury occurs. Since bone and soft tissue resistance to injury decreases with age, elderly vehicle occupants are at increased risk of injury; this trend reaches statistical significance in the 7th decade. The location of injury depends on which structures strike which car component and the severity depends on the speed and energy of the collision as well as timing of human contact to car structures. In a frontal collision an occupant continues to move forward as the vehicle stops. Forward motion of the occupant is arrested as the person connects either with the seatbelt or with anterior car structures, if unrestrained. Initial impact points are often lower extremities, resulting in fractures of the ankle, around the knee, or fracture of the femur. There are many factors that contribute to the amount of force transferred to specific anatomical structures including change in velocity at impact, timing of impact, degree of compartment intrusion, configuration of occupant and safety devices Change in velocity at time of impact is closely associated with severity of injury as well as incidence of lower extremity injury. The effect of timing is illustrated in the different degree of injury sustained when knee contact with instrument panel occurs during deceleration when the instrument panel may still be moving forward causing the localized contact velocity to be lower than impacts that occur once the car has stopped moving. Occupant factors, such as age, gender, height and BMI also contribute to type and severity of injury. Height appears to be an important factor in pattern of injury; tall occupants (and males) sustain more knee, thigh or hip injuries while shorter (and female) occupants tend to sustain more foot and ankle injuries. Elderly occupants are at increased risk of injury. There are studies that indicate that high BMI's are associated with increased severity of lower extremity injury.

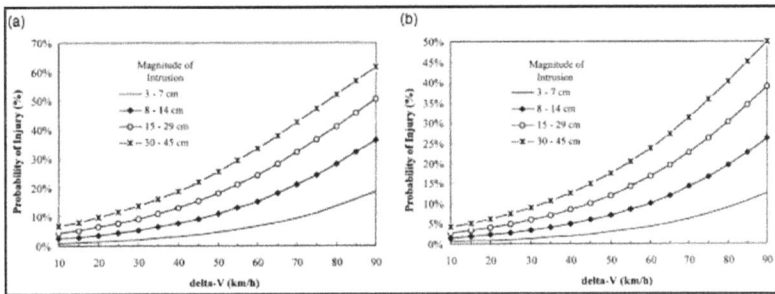

Injury risk in a frontal MVC is related to magnitude of car intrusion and delta-V for both female (a) and male (b) occupants.

A typical dashboard injury pattern is often initiated by knee impact, usually on the instrument panel. This occurs most frequently in unrestrained occupants with or without airbag deployment. Force to the knee from the dashboard or instrument panel can result in knee laceration, patellar fracture, distal femur fracture, and proximal tibia fracture and forces can be transmitted through the femur to cause femoral shaft fractures, proximal femur fractures, acetabular or pelvic fractures, and posterior hip dislocation. The risks for hip/pelvis injuries are generally greater than the risk for knee and thigh injuries at all crash severities and the right hip is more often injured than the left in forward-moving crashes, likely due to the effects of braking and bracing on occupant position and on muscle tension. Hip/pelvis fractures occur at lower impact force when the hip is flexed or adducted prior to impact; hip tolerance decreases approximately 1.8% for each degree of adduction from neutral and approximately 1% for each degree of flexion. In an unrestrained driver, the body continues moving forward after the vehicle has stopped and the head, cervical spine and torso impact the windshield and steering wheel. During a lateral impact the occupant is accelerated away from the side of the vehicle that was struck and common injuries include lateral compression pelvic fracture, pulmonary contusion and intraabdominal solid organ injury.

The other primary mechanism for lower extremity injury during a motor vehicle collision is impact caused by pedal interaction and toe pan intrusion. One specific fracture that is well described is calcaneus or malleous fracture of the foot secondary to being forced against the brake pedal by the weight of the occupant or in combination with the floor pan of the car crushing into the space where the foot resides. When the Achilles tendon resists dorsiflexion and the brake causes dorsiflexion, a three-point bending load occurs on the calcaneus with the posterior facet of the talus functioning as a fulcrum. This leads to a specific fracture pattern referred to as the tongue-toe calcaneous fracture pattern. Foot inversion or eversion in combination with compression force created by the brake pedal leads to malleolus fracture. High-heeled shoes have been shown to alter foot and ankle biomechanics leading to increased instability and injury during an MVC. The effect of height on pattern of injury may be a reflection of leg position and may be related to the fact that shorter people sit closer to the steering wheel and reach for foot pedals, while taller people sit farther back with their knees closer to the level of the instrument panel.

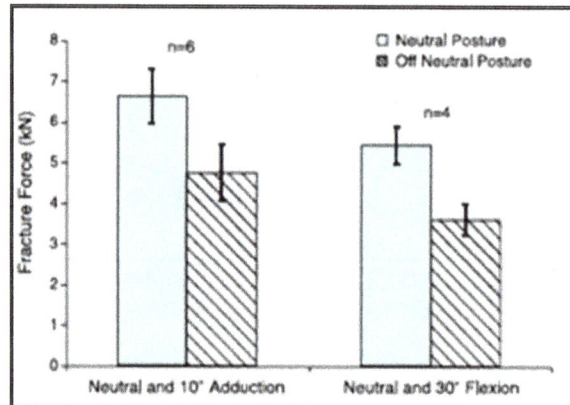

Hip/pelvis fx occurs at lower impact force when the hip is flexed or adducted prior to impact.

Many safety systems, including seat belts, air bags, and vehicle deformation, take advantage of the fact that increasing time over which decelerations are applied to the passenger compartment decreases force experienced by the occupants. The concept of a "crumple zone" is based on this effect. Newer car designs provide an average of 2 ft of crushable car body, as well as steering mechanisms that collapse, which functions to increase deceleration time and also to dissipate a component of the energy by deformation. Early goals of impact biomechanics and development of safety technology focused on decreasing mortality and head and thorax injuries to the extent that lower extremities are now the regions most likely to sustain injuries in frontal MVCs (Rupp & Schneider, 2004). These injuries are of substantial concern because they now account for up to 40% of treatment cost and nearly half of patients report significant long-term disability.

Seat belts have had the single largest effect on reducing MVC-related mortality and injury, including extremity injury, decreasing fatalities by approximately 45-50%. Seat belts increase deceleration time of the occupant via stretching of seat belt webbing and they distribute forces more uniformly on the body. There are multiple improvements in seatbelt technology that contribute to this effect. Pre-tensioners remove slack from the seatbelt upon detection of crash condition. Load limiters limits force imparted to the occupant by the seatbelt during the crash event by allowing the seatbelt webbing to yield when forces reach the set level. Web clamps lock the webbing to prevent or to minimize shoulder belt spool-out.

Air bags are universally present in all new cars due to federal regulations, and it is well documented that they reduce risk of MVC-related mortality by 4-25%. However, there is controversy regarding their effect on non-fatal injuries, particularly musculoskeletal injury. Air bag deployment without seat belt restraint is associated with increased incidence of lower extremity injury and some data suggests that air bag deployment together with seat belt restraint is also associated with increased incidence of lower extremity injury. A possible contributing factor to the increased incidence of lower extremity injury is a "submarining" effect in which the pelvis and lower extremities are shifted under the airbag and down the seat into the knee bolster and floor of the car. Lower extremity trauma leads to significant impairments in function, and may be the most frequent cause of permanent disability after motor vehicle collision. Improvement in safety systems directed at preventing lower extremity injury will be critical in the future. There is now increased interest in "knee bolster airbags" which could reduce the negative impact of airbags on lower extremity injury and in "smart air bags". These would be able to accurately sense the crash pulse, deploy in a graded fashion depending on the occupant size and weight, and deploy only when truly necessary.

Anterior Cruciate Ligament (ACL) Tear

Nearly 75% of ACL injuries are non-contact and occur as a result of self-initiated movement usually during athletic activities. The mechanism of injury is based on the anatomy of the knee. The ACL is a fibrous connective tissue that attaches the posterior aspect of the femur to the anterior aspect of the tibia. It courses anteriorly, medially and distally as it runs from femur to tibia. The primary function of the ACL is to limit anterior translation of the tibia relative to the femur.

ACL injuries are usually associated with decelerating and changing direction; often ACL injuries are caused by an internal twisting of the tibia relative to the femur or combination of torque and compression during a landing. Despite intense study of the ACL injury during the past three decades, the exact mechanism of injury is not known. ACL injury occurs when an excessive tension force is applied to the ACL. It has also been noted that in 96% of ACL tears, an opposing player is within close proximity, which could cause an alteration in the players' coordination leading to dangerous leg positions. There is some controversy as to how this force occurs, but based on recent studies, it is likely that an axial compressive force acting on the posterior tibial slope contributes to many ACL tears. This axial force results in posterior displacement of the femoral condyle on the tibial plateau, which applies tension to the ACL. Boden et al found that subjects who experienced an ACL tear initially came into contact with the ground with their hindfoot or with their foot flat (the "provocative" landing position), whereas control subjects landed on the forefoot. It appears that normally, during landing, the foot, ankle, knee and hip joints work to dampen ground reaction forces. However, when subjects come into contact with the ground with the hindfoot or with their foot flat, the foot, ankle, and calf muscles are not able to absorb ground reaction forces, and the leg is converted into a two-segment column (above and below the knee), and the knee ends up absorbing a large component of the loading force. Additionally, under normal circumstances, as the calf muscles contract during absorption of ground-reaction forces, they produce a flexion force on the knee, activating the normal knee absorption mechanics. In the absence of calf muscle contraction, the knee may abduct or internally rotate rather than flex. Additionally, higher hip flexion angle at landing places the torso farther posterior to the knee, requiring that the quadriceps muscle must be activating during landing. The quadriceps muscle force provides anterior shear force on the proximal tibia which increases ACL strain. Knee abduction (or knee valgus) also may play a role, particularly in female athletes, by potentially reducing the compression force threshold needed to produce ACL injury. However, it may also be that valgus collapse is the result of the ACL being torn rather than a cause.

References

- Overview-of-the-skeletal-system, boundless-ap: courses.lumenlearning.com, Retrieved 17 February, 2019

- Neuromuscular-system: healthdirect.gov.au, Retrieved 14 June, 2019

- Tözeren, Aydın (2000). Human Body Dynamics: Classical Mechanics and Human Movement. Springer. pp. 6–10. ISBN 0-387-98801-7

- Musculoskeletal-injuries- 5241: safeopedia.com, Retrieved 25 January, 2019

- Biomechanics-of-musculoskeletal-injury, biomechanics-in-applications: intechopen.com, Retrieved 18 May, 2019

3

Concepts in Biomechanics

Some of the concepts of biomechanics include aggregate modulus, limits of stability, ground reaction force, Hill's muscle model, Moens-Korteweg equation, gait cycle, functional spinal unit, Womersley number, Tinetti test, etc. This chapter closely examines these key concepts of biomechanics to provide an extensive understanding of the subject.

BALANCE

Balance refers to an individual's ability to maintain their line of gravity within their Base of support (BOS). It can also be described as the ability to maintain equilibrium, where equilibrium can be defined as any condition in which all acting forces are cancelled by each other resulting in a stable balanced system.

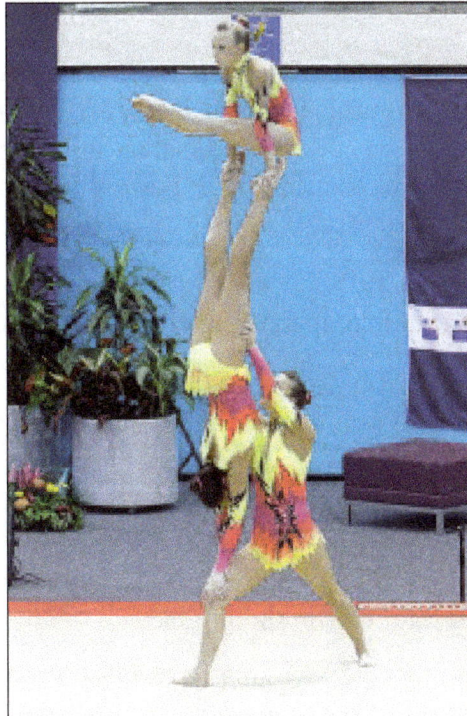

In literature, the balance term has been used synonymously with:

- Postural Control.

- Postural Stability.

- Equilibrium.

Balance Systems

The following system provides input regarding the body's equilibrium and thus maintains balance:

- Somatosensory / Proprioceptive System.

- Vestibular System.

- Visual System.

The Central Nervous System receives feedback about the body orientation from these three main sensory systems and integrates this sensory feedback and subsequently generates a corrective, stabilizing torque by selectively activating muscles. In normal condition, healthy subjects rely 70% on somatosensory information and 20% Vestibular & 10% on Vision on firm surface but change to 60% vestibular information, 30% Vision & 10% somatosensory on unstable surface.

Somatosensory System

Proprioceptive information from spino-cerebellar pathways, processed unconsciously in the cerebellum, are required to control postural balance. Proprioceptive information has the shortest time delays, with monosynaptic pathways that can process information as quickly as 40–50 ms and hence the major contributor for postural control in normal conditions.

Vestibular System

The vestibular system generates compensatory responses to head motion via:

- Postural responses (Vestibulo Spinal Reflex): Keep the body upright and prevent falls when the body is unexpectedly knocked off balance.

- Ocular-motor responses (Vestibulo Ocular Reflex): Allows the eyes to remain steadily focused while the head is in motion.

- Visceral responses (Vestibulo Colic Reflex): Help keep the head and neck centred, steady, and upright on the shoulders.

To achieve this the vestibular system measures head rotation and head acceleration through semicircular canals and otolith organs (utricule and sacule).

Visual System

For non-impaired individuals under normal conditions the contribution of visual system to postural control is partially redundant as the visual information has the longer time delays as long as 150-200 ms. Friedrich et al. observed that adults with visual disorders were able to adapt peripheral, vestibular, somatosensoric perception and cerebellar processing to compensate their visual information deficit and to provide good postural control. In addition, Peterka found that adults with bilateral vestibular deficits can enhance their visual and proprioceptive information even more than healthy adults in order to reach an effective postural stability. The influence of moving visual fields on postural stability depends on the characteristics of the visual environment, and of the support surface, including the size of the base of support, its rigidity or compliance.

Static and Dynamic Balance

Balance can be classified in to:

- Static Balance: It is the ability to maintain the body in some fixed posture. Static balance is the ability to maintain postural stability and orientation with centre of mass over the base of support and body at rest.

- Dynamic Balance: Defining dynamic postural stability is more challenging, Dynamic balance is the ability to transfer the vertical projection of the centre of gravity around the supporting base of support. Dynamic balance is the ability to maintain postural stability and orientation with centre of mass over the base of support while the body parts are in motion.

Mechanisms

The mechanisms involved in static balance were best summarized by Bannister. He noted that normal standing required:

- Sufficient power in the muscles of the lower limbs and trunk to maintain the body erect.

- Normal postural sensibility to convey information concerning position.

- Normal impulses from the vestibular labyrinth concerning position.

- A central coordinating mechanism, the chief part of which is the vermis of the cerebellum.

- The activity of higher centers concerned in the willed maintenance of posture.

With this mechanisms the dynamic balance requirements can be inferred as:

- Sufficient power in the muscles of the body to maintain movement and stability.

- Normal postural sensibility to convey information regarding movement.

- Normal impulses from the vestibular system and visual system concering movement and environment.

- Central coordinating mechanism including cerebellum and basal ganglia.

- The activity of higher centers concerned in the willed/ involuntary maintenance of movement and stability.

Correlation between Static and Dynamic Balance

A study by Sell TC examined the relationship and differences between static and dynamic postural stability in healthy, physically active adults. Static postural stability was measured by a single-leg standing task and dynamic postural stability was measured by a single-leg landing task using the Dynamic Postural Stability Index. The author concludes that there was a lack of a correlation between static and dynamic measures. However, the increase in difficulty during dynamic measures indicates differences in the type and magnitude of challenge imposed by the different postural stability tasks.

The lack of correlation between the two different conditions is likely due to the challenge imposed on the systems necessary for maintenance of postural stability. Maintenance of postural stability during both dynamic and static conditions involves establishing an equilibrium between destabilizing and stabilizing forces and requires sensory information derived from vision, the vestibular systems, and somatosensory feedback.

Management of Balance in Specific Conditions

Parkinson's

Parkinson's is a progressive neurodegenerative disease. It's often characterized by tremor, bradykinesia, postural instability and rigidity. Most frequently, patients have gait impairments, difficulty in linking movements together smoothly and episodes of freezing. The sum of these problems, together with balance disturbances lead to an increased incidence of falls.

The physiotherapist is a member of the multidisciplinary team, with the purpose of maximising functional ability and minimising secondary complications. Physiotherapy for Parkinson's disease focuses on: transfers, posture, upper limb function, balance, gait, and physical capacity. The therapist uses cueing strategies, cognitive movement strategies and exercise to maintain or increase independence, safety, and quality of life. Sensory cueing strategies such as auditory, tactile, and visual cues have often been used to help walking in PD.

Cognitive Movement Strategies

Cognitive movement strategies are used to improve transfers. Complex and automatic activities are divided into separate elements consisting of relatively simple movement components. By doing this, the person has to think consciously about his movements. Try to avoid dual tasking during complex automatic ADL. Furthermore, the movement or activity will be practiced and rehearsed in the mind. It is important that movements are not performed automatically; performance has to be consciously controlled Example: Sit to stand.

- Hands on chair.

- Place feet correctly.

- Move forward.

- Flex trunk.

- Rise up from chair.

Cueing Strategies

The performance of automatic and repetitive movements of patients with Parkinson's is disturbed as a result of fundamental problems of internal control. That's why cues are used to complete or replace this reduced internal control. Cues can be generated internally or externally. Rhythmical recurring cues are given as a continuous rhythmical stimulus, which can serve as a control mechanism for walking.

- Auditory (moves on music/ walkman, singing, counting).

- Visual (p follows another person, walks over stripes on the floor or over stripes he projects to himself with a laserpen).

- Tactile(p taps his hip or leg).

The Physical Therapeutic Intervention Goals Apply to the Phase Addressed

Early phase: patients have no or little limitations. Goals of the therapeutic intervention are:

- Prevention of inactivity.

- Prevention of fear to move/to fall.

- Preserving/ improving physical capacity.

Mid phase: more severe symptoms; performance of activities become restricted, problems with balance and an increased risk of falls, Problems:

- Transfers.

- Body posture.

- Reaching and grasping.

- Balance.

- Gait.

Late phase: patients are confined to a wheelchair or bed. The treatment goal in this phase is to preserve vital functions and to prevent complications, such as pressure sores and contractures.

Elderly

Balance training can also be used in the elderly. Falls of elderly, due to poor balance, has important clinical and economical costs and intervention. For this reason, it is interesting to search for possibilities to reduce these costs, such as the use of balance training.

In 2011, weak evidence has been found for the effectiveness of several exercises in improving clinical balance outcomes in elderly:

- Gait.

- Balance.

- Co-ordination and functional tasks.

- Strengthening exercise.

- But evidence for the effect of computerized balance programs or vibration plates is insufficient.

To keep the therapy adherence up it is best to look for an approach with a 'fun factor'. Some examples:

- Music-based multitask exercise program: Basic exercises consisted of walking in time to the music and responding to changes in the music's rhythmic patterns. Exercises involved a wide range of movements and challenged the balance control system mainly by requiring multidirectional weight shifting, walk-and-turn sequences, and exaggerated upper body movements when walking and standing.

- Balance training using a virtual-reality system: In contrast to the review of 2011, in 2013 it was found an effective method to train the balance in older fallers. This method is intended to complete, not replace, other fall prevention programs.

- Tai chi: Tai chi has been proven to be an economic and effective way for training balance in older people. To ameliorate balance in elderly it isn't enough to just follow a conventional exercise intervention (including muscle strengthening, stretching and aerobic exercises, and health education). Besides this it is better to also include static and dynamic balance exercises.

Examples of static balance exercises: Squats, two-leg stance and one-leg stance.

Examples of dynamic exercises: Jogging end to end, sideways walking or running with crossovers, forward walking or running in a zigzag line, backward walking or running in zigzag line.

Nevertheless to improve balance core strength training is an important element. The benefit is this therapy can be both given in a group setting or in individual fall preventive interventions.

BASE OF SUPPORT

The base of support (BOS) refers to the area beneath an object or person that includes every point of contact that the object or person makes with the supporting surface. These points of contact may be body parts e.g. feet or hands, or they may include things like crutches or the chair a person is sitting in.

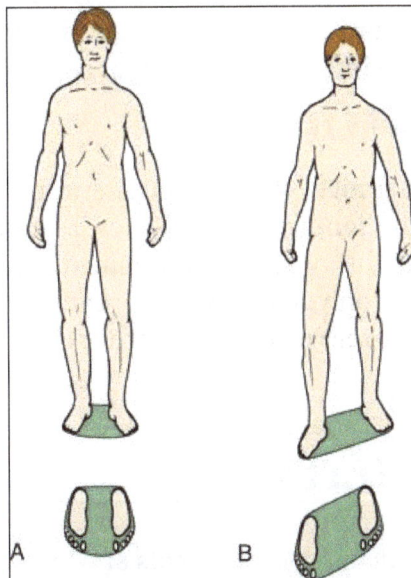

Significance

The BOS is an important concept to understand an individual's ability to Balance, as balance is defined as the ability to maintain the line of gravity (passing through the Centre of Gravity) within the BOS.

In gait, the base of support has been defined as the horizontal stride width during the double-support phase when both feet are in contact with the ground and the whole-body center of gravity (CG) remains within the BOS. A wide base of support (BOS) has long been believed to be a hallmark of unsteady gait.

Clinical Implication

- A decreased stride width is found to closely correlate with fall frequency and dynamic stability.

- The majority of the gait cycle is spent in single leg support during which the BOS is minimized to the width of the supporting foot.

- Thus, when a patient is tried for gait, the wider base of support by means of walking aids such as walker, crutches, cane, etc is provided to acquire more stability. As the condition of the patient improves, the BOS can be reduced.

AGGREGATE MODULUS

In relation to biomechanics, the aggregate modulus (Ha) is a measurement of the stiffness of a material at equilibrium when fluid has ceased flowing through it. The aggregate modulus can be calculated from Young's modulus (E) and the Poisson ratio (v).

$$H a = E (1 - v) / [(1 + v) (1 - 2 v)]$$

The aggregate modulus of a similar specimen is determined from a unidirectional *deformational* testing configuration, i.e., the only non-zero strain component is E_{11}, as opposed to the Young's modulus, which is determined from a unidirectional *loading* testing configuration, i.e., the only non-zero stress component is, say, in the e_1 direction. In this test, the only non-zero component of the stress tensor is T_{11}.

LIMITS OF STABILITY

Limits of Stability (LoS) are defined as the points at which the center of gravity (CoG) approaches the limits of the base of support (BoS) and a correction strategy is required to return the center of mass (CoM) to within the BoS."In other words, LoS is the amount of maximum excursion an individual is able to intentionally cover in any direction without losing his/her balance or taking a step. The normal sway angle in the antero-posterior direction and medio-lateral direction is approximately 12.5° and 16° respectively. This area of stable swaying is often referred to as the 'Cone of Stability'. The limits of this cone of stability keep changing constantly depending on the task being performed.

Once the CoG moves outside the BoS, the individual must step or grasp an external device in-order to maintain his balance and refrain himself from falling.

These stability limits are perceived rather than the physiological, i.e. it is the readiness of the subject to change their COG position.

Clinical Significance

LoS is a reliable variable of stability that provides important information about voluntary motor control in the dynamic state. LoS helps assess balance in the dynamic state by instantaneously tracking the change in COM velocity and COM position. The LoS measures postural instability while screening for individuals who are at a higher risk of falling. Individuals with decreased LoS have an increased risk of falling when they shift their bodyweight forward, backward or from side to side and hence are more prone to injuries.

A restricted LoS significantly influences the ability to react to perturbations in balance control testing. This reduction in LoS may be because of weakness of the ankle and foot muscles, musculoskeletal problems of the lower limb, and/or an internal perception of the subject to resist larger displacements. These impairments may help physicians to correlate with the medical examination findings and serve as an important outcome measure for rehabilitation of these specific underlying body impairments. From a clinical perspective, an individual who performs complex mobility tasks can function without support, and is better able to tolerate environmental challenges.

Possible Causes of LOS Impairment

- Impaired cognitive processing usually due to aging leading to attention deficits.
- Neuromuscular Impairments such as bradykinesia, ataxia, or poor motor control.
- Musculoskeletal Impairements such as weakness, limited ROM, pain.
- Emotional Overlay like fear or anxiety.
- Aphysiology (exaggeration or poor effort).

Limits of Stability Testing

Various tools such as the Functional Reach Test (FRT) and Limits Of Stability (LOS) test have been used to assess LoS.

- FRT: This is the conventional test used to assess balance and LoS in the forward direction. FRT is inexpensive and easy to use. The drawback of this test is that it assess balance issues in a standing posture where the feet are in a static position and measures LoS only in the forward direction.

- LOS: This is a more sophisticated tool than FRT used to measure balance under multi-directional conditions. The subject is asked to stand on force plates and intentionally shift his body weight in the cued direction.

Parameters Measured in LOS Test

- Reaction Time (RT): The time taken by an individual to start shifting his center of gravity (COG) from the static position after the cue, measured in seconds.

- Movement Velocity (MVL): The average speed at which the COG shifts.

- EndPoint Excursions (EPE): The distance willingly covered by the subject in his very first attempt towards the target, expressed as a percentage.

- Maximum Excursions (MXE): The amount of distance the subject actually covered or moved his COG.

- Directional Control (DCL): A comparison between the amount of movement demonstrated in the desired direction, i.e. towards the target, to the amount of external movement in the opposite direction of the target, expressed as a percentage.

Interpretation of LOS Results

The capability of moving around without falling is necessary for activities of daily living (ADL's). Patients exhibiting delay in the reaction time, decreased movement velocity, restricted LoS boundary or cone of stability, or uncontrolled CoG movement are at a higher risk of falling. A delayed reaction time suggests that the individual might have problems in cognitive processing. Reduced movement velocities are indicate high-level of central nervous system deficits. Reduced Endpoint excursions, excessively larger maximum excursions and poor directional control are all indicative of motor control abnormalities.

A LOS scores close to 100 represents no sway and hence reduced risk of fall, while scores close to 0 imply a higher risk of falling.

Validity and Reliability of LOS

The LOS test has been validated for use across multiple patient populations that include community dwelling elderly, neurological disorders, and back and knee injuries. A study conducted by Wernick-Robinson and collaborators on the test retest reliability suggest that the amount of distance covered in the functional reach test alone cannot be an adequate measure of dynamic balance. It also suggests that for a better evaluation of postural control, additional assessment of movement strategies is indispensable.

Another study done by Brouwer et al. also claimed that LOS was a reliable measure for balance testing in healthy populations.

Functional Impact and Implications of LOS

The capability of moving around without falling is necessary for activities of daily living (ADL's). Instability during weight-shifting activities, or the inability to perform certain weight transfer tasks such as bending forward to take objects from a shelf, leaning backward to rinse hair in the shower, etc. can result from a restricted LoS boundary. The ability to voluntarily move the COG to positions within the Limits of Stability (LOS) with control is fundamental to independence and safety in mobility tasks such as reaching for objects, transitioning from seated to standing positions (or standing to seated) and walking. The LoS can be indicative of fall risks in the elderly, individuals with movement disorders and in neurologically impaired populations. The ability to voluntarily move the COG to positions within the Limits of Stability (LOS) with control is fundamental to independence and safety in mobility tasks such as reaching for objects, transitioning from seated to standing positions (or standing to seated) and walking.

CENTER OF PRESSURE

In biomechanics, center of pressure (CoP) is the term given to the point of application of the ground reaction force vector. The ground reaction force vector represents the sum of all forces acting between a physical object and its supporting surface. Analysis of the center of pressure is common in studies on human postural control and gait. It is thought that changes in motor control may be reflected in changes in the center of pressure. In biomechanical studies, the effect of some experimental condition on movement execution will regularly be quantified by alterations in the center of pressure.

The center of pressure is not a static outcome measure. For instance, during human walking, the center of pressure is near the heel at the time of heelstrike and moves anteriorly throughout the step, being located near the toes at toe-off. For this reason, analysis of the center of pressure will need to take into account the dynamic nature of the signal. In the scientific literature various methods for the analysis of center of pressure time series have been proposed.

Measuring CoP

CoP measurements are commonly gathered through the use of a force plate. A force plate gathers data in the anterior-posterior direction (forward and backward), the medial-lateral direction (side-to-side) and the vertical direction, as well as moments about all 3 axes. Together, these can be used to calculate the position of the center of pressure relative to the origin of the force plate.

Relationship to Balance

CoP and center of gravity (CoG) are both related to balance in that they are dependent on the position of the body with respect to the supporting surface. Center of gravity is subject to change based on posture. Center of pressure is the location on the supporting surface where the resultant vertical force vector would act if it could be considered to have a single point of application.

A shift of CoP is an indirect measure of postural sway and thus a measure of a person's ability to maintain balance. All people would sway in the anterior-posterior direction (forward and backward) and the medial-lateral direction (side-to-side) when they are simply standing still. This comes as a result of small contractions of muscles in your body to maintain an upright position. An increase in sway is not necessarily an indicator of poorer balance so much as it is an indicator of decreased neuromuscular control, although it has been noted that postural sway is a precursor to a fall.

GROUND REACTION FORCE

The ground reaction force is equal in magnitude and opposite in direction to the force that the body exerts on the supporting surface through the foot.

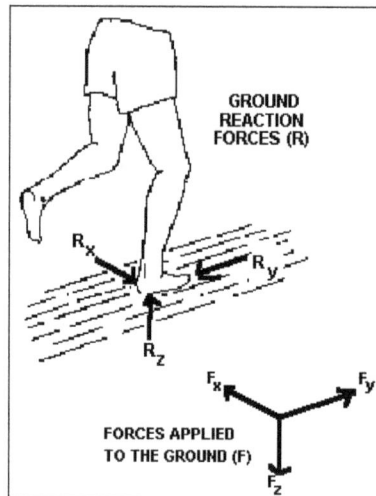

The ground reaction force vector (GRFV) passes upward from the foot and produces movement at each lower extremity joint. We can visualize the GRFV by studying laboratory investigations of normal gait that employ force plates to measure the GRFV's three-dimensional orientation.

The GRFV differs from a "gravity line," which is a vector that extends vertically from the center of gravity of a static body. Instead, the GRFV is a "reflection of the total mass-times-acceleration product of all body segments and therefore represents the total of all net muscle and gravitational forces acting at each instant of time over the stance period".

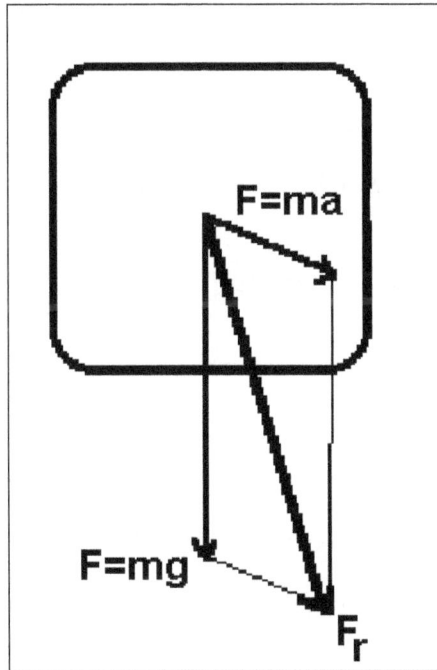

$F=mg$ designates the vector that represents the force of gravity acting on the object.

$F=ma$ designates the vector that represents the instantaneous inertial force acting on the object. In this diagram, inertial forces accelerate the body toward downward and to the right.

Vector (F_r) is the resultant or sum of the gravitational and inertial forces.

In contact with a stable surface like the ground, vector F_r represents a force that is opposed by a ground reaction force of equal magnitude. Because the ground reaction force is equal and opposite, its vector's line of application is the same as that of F_r, and it has the same effect on the body and its joints.

The GRFV combines both gravity's effect on the body and the effects of the body's movement and acceleration (change of velocity) in three planes of reference. This makes the

GRFV especially suitable for the study of gait, during which the body's various masses undergo complex accelerations.

Sophisticated gait analysis equipment can generate a visible force vector on an oscilloscope screen and superimpose it simultaneously on a photograph of a gait subject. Visualizing ground reaction forces helps us understand their effects on the body during walking, and permits us to predict muscle activity using a simple model:

$$M_{mm} = -M_{GRF}$$

We can predict muscle activity quite accurately if we take the view that the ground reaction force (GRF) and the muscles (mm) produce equal and opposite moments (M) around each joint.

Measuring the Ground Reaction Forces

The most direct and effective way to measure ground reaction forces (GRF) is using a force plate.

In biomechanics force plates are applied to:

- Characterize walking.

- Characterize running.

- Characterize jumping.

Benefit of Measuring Ground Reaction Forces

GRFs are one of the most often analyzed biomechanical measures and help characterize human movements. Measuring GRFs plays an important role in the areas of:

- Sports performance analysis.

- Rehabilitation.

- Products ergonomics.

- Clinical research.

HILL'S MUSCLE MODEL

In biomechanics, Hill's muscle model refers to either Hill's equations for tetanized muscle contraction or to the 3-element model. They were derived by the famous physiologist Archibald Vivian Hill.

Equation to Tetanized Muscle

This is a popular state equation applicable to skeletal muscle that has been stimulated to show Tetanic contraction. It relates tension to velocity with regard to the internal thermodynamics. The equation is:

$$(v + b)(F + a) = b(F_0 + a)$$

Where,

- F is the tension (or load) in the muscle.

- v is the velocity of contraction.

- F_0 is the maximum isometric tension (or load) generated in the muscle.

- a coefficient of shortening heat.

- $b = a \cdot v_0 / F_0$.

- v_0 is the maximum velocity, when $F = 0$.

Although Hill's equation looks very much like the van der Waals equation, the former has units of energy dissipation, while the latter has units of energy. Hill's equation demonstrates that the relationship between F and v is hyperbolic. Therefore, the higher the load applied to the muscle, the lower the contraction velocity. Similarly, the higher the contraction velocity, the lower the tension in the muscle. This hyperbolic form has been found to fit the empirical constant only during isotonic contractions near resting length.

The muscle tension decreases as the shortening velocity increases. This feature has been attributed to two main causes. The major appears to be the loss in tension as the cross bridges in the contractile element and then reform in a shortened condition. The second cause appears to be the fluid viscosity in both the contractile element and the connective tissue. Whichever the cause of loss of tension, it is a viscous friction and can therefore be modeled as a fluid damper.

Three-element Model

The three-element Hill muscle model is a representation of the muscle mechanical response. The model is constituted by a contractile element (CE) and two non-linear spring elements, one in series (SE) and another in parallel (PE). The active force of the contractile element comes from the force generated by the actin and myosin cross-bridges at the sarcomere level. It is fully extensible when inactive but capable of shortening when activated. The connective tissues (fascia, epimysium, perimysium and endomysium) that surround the contractile element influences the muscle's force-length curve. The parallel element represents the passive force of these connective tissues and has a soft tissue mechanical behavior. The parallel element is responsible for the muscle passive behavior when it is stretched, even when the contractile element is not activated. The series element represents the tendon and the intrinsic elasticity of the myofilaments. It also has a soft tissue response and provides energy storing mechanism.

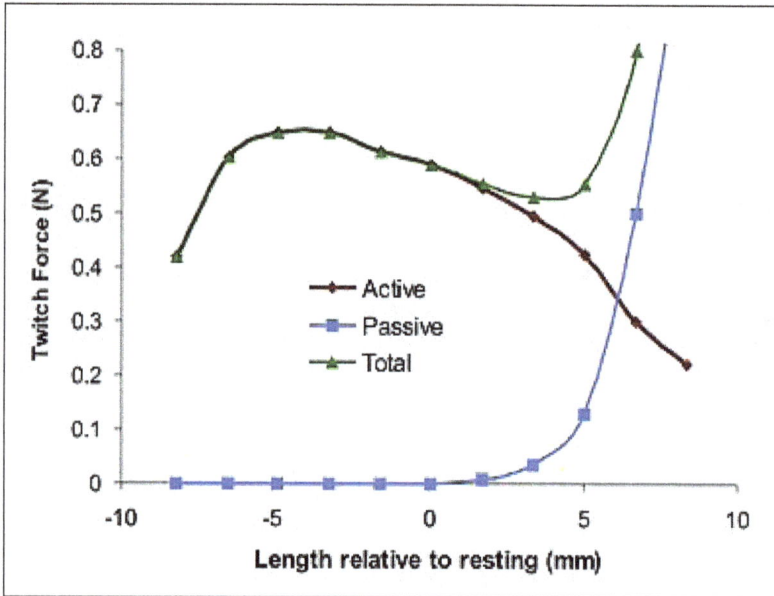

Muscle length vs Force. In Hill's muscle model the active and passive forces are respectively F_{CE} and F_{PE}.

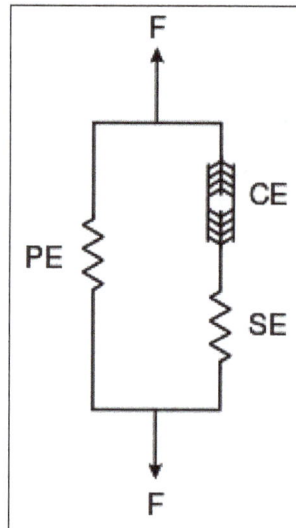

Hill's elastic muscle model. F: Force; CE: Contractile Element; SE: Series Element; PE: Parallel Element.

The net force-length characteristics of a muscle is a combination of the force-length characteristics of both active and passive elements. The forces in the contractile element, in the series element and in the parallel element, F_{CE}, F_{SE} and F_{PE}, respectively, satisfy

$$F = F_{PE} + F_{SE} \quad \text{and} \quad F_{CE} = F_{SE}.$$

On the other hand, the muscle length L and the lengths L_{CE}, L_{SE} and L_{PE} of those elements satisfy:

$$L = L_{PE} \quad \text{and} \quad L = L_{CE} + L_{SE}.$$

During isometric contractions the series elastic component is under tension and therefore is stretched a finite amount. Because the overall length of the muscle is kept constant, the stretching of the series element can only occur if there is an equal shortening of the contractile element itself.

Viscoelasticity

Muscles present viscoelasticity, therefore a viscous damper may be included in the model, when the dynamics of the second-order critically damped twitch is regarded. One common model for muscular viscosity is an exponential form damper, where

$$F_D = k(\dot{L}_D)^a$$

is added to the model's global equation, whose k and a are constants.

MOENS-KORTEWEG EQUATION

In biomechanics, the Moens–Korteweg equation models the relationship between wave speed or pulse wave velocity (PWV) and the incremental elastic modulus of the arterial wall or its distensibility. The equation was derived independently by Adriaan Isebree Moens and Diederik Korteweg. It is derived from Newton's second law of motion, using some simplifying assumptions, and reads:

$$PWV = \sqrt{\frac{E_{inc} \cdot h}{2r\rho}}$$

The Moens–Korteweg equation states that PWV is proportional to the square root of the incremental elastic modulus, (E_{inc}), of the vessel wall given constant ratio of wall thickness, h, to vessel radius, r, and blood density, ρ, assuming that the artery wall is isotropic and experiences isovolumetric change with pulse pressure.

LINES OF NON-EXTENSION

In the field of biomechanics, the lines of non-extension are notional lines running across the human body along which body movement causes neither stretching or contraction.

Discovered by Arthur Iberall in work beginning in the 1940s, as part of research into space suit design, they have been further developed by Dava Newman in the development of the Space Activity Suit.

They were originally mapped by Iberall by drawing a series of circles over a portion of the body and then watching their deformations as the wearer walked around or performed various tasks. The circles deform into ellipses as the skin stretches over the moving musculature, and these deformations were recorded. After a huge number of such measurements the data is then examined to find all of the possible deformations of the circles, and more importantly, the non-moving points on them where the original circle and the deformed ellipse intersect (at four points per circle). By mapping these points over the entire body, a series of lines are produced.

These lines may then be used to direct the placement of tension elements in a spacesuit to enable constant suit pressure regardless of the motion of the body.

GAIT CYCLE

A (bipedal) gait cycle is the time period or sequence of events or movements during locomotion in which one foot contacts the ground to when that same foot again contacts the ground, and involves propulsion of the centre of gravity in the direction of motion.

The gait cycle is a repetitive pattern involving steps and strides. A step is one single step, a stride is a whole gait cycle. The step time is the time between heel strike of one leg and heel strike of the contra-lateral leg. Step width can be described as the medio-lateral space between the two feet.

There are some differences between the gait and run cycle - the gait cycle is one third longer in time, the ground reaction force is smaller in the gait cycle (so the load is lower), and the velocity is much higher. In running, there is also just one stance phase while in stepping there are two. Shock absorption is also much larger in comparison to walking. This explains why runners have more overload injuries.

The sequences for walking that occur may be summarised as follows:

- Registration and activation of the gait command within the central nervous system.

- Transmission of the gait systems to the peripheral nervous system.

- Contraction of muscles.

- Generation of several forces.

- Regulation of joint forces and moments across synovial joints and skeletal segments.

- Generation of ground reaction forces.

Classification of the gait cycle involves two main phases: the stance phase and the swing phase. The stance phase occupies 60% of the gait cycle while the swing phase occupies only 40% of it. Gait involves a combination of open and close chain activities. A more detailed classification of gait recognises six phases:

- Heel strike.

- Foot flat.

- Mid-stance.

- Heel-off.

- Toe-off.

- Mid-swing.

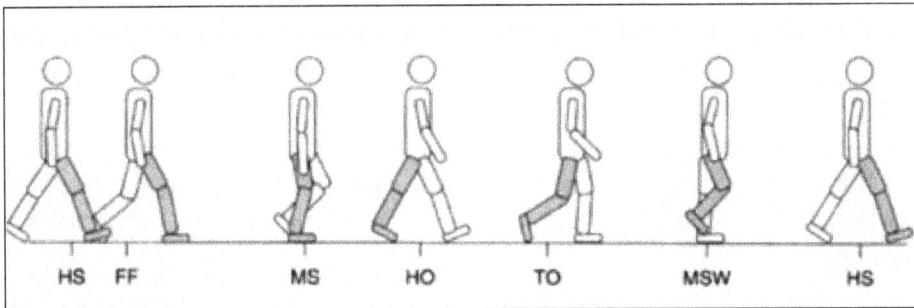

An alternative classification of gait involves the following eight phases:

- Initial contact.

- Loading response.

- Midstance.

- Terminal stance.

- Pre swing.

- Initial swing.

- Mid swing.

- Late swing.

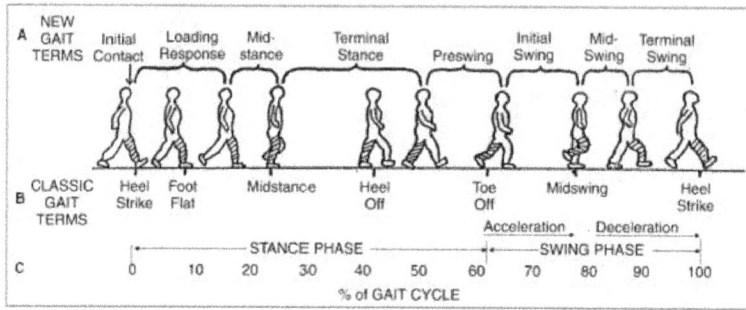

Demos, Gait analysis.

- Stance phase begins with the heel strike. This is the moment when the heel begins to touch the ground but the toes do not yet touch. In the midstance phase, we can see settlement of the foot at the lateral border. During the change from mid-stance to toe-off stance, the 5 metacarpophalanges contract. The toe-off phase is also named the propulsive phase.

- Swing phase begins, when the stance phase ends, This phase is the phase between the toe-off phase and the heel strike phase. In the swing-phase we can recognise two extra phases - acceleration and declaration The acceleration phase goes from toe-off to midswing, while deceleration goes from midswing to heel strike. In the acceleration phase, the swing leg makes an accelerated forward movement with the goal of propelling the bodyweight forward. The declaration phase brakes the velocity of this forward body movement in order to place your foot down with control. Between these two phases, the mid-swing phase occurs. In this phase, both feet are under the body, with the heel next to each other.

Phases of the Gait Cycle

Heel Strike

Also known as initial contact, is a short period which begins the moment the foot touches the ground and is the first phase of double support. 30° flexion of the hip and full extension in the knee is observed. The ankle moves from a neutral (supinated 5°) position into plantar flexion. After this, knee flexion (5°) begins and increases, just as the plantar flexion of the heel increased. The plantar flexion is allowed by eccentric contraction of the tibialis anterior, extension of the knee is caused by a contraction of the quadriceps, flexion is caused by a contraction of the hamstrings, and the flexion of the hip is caused by the contraction of the rectus femoris.

Foot Flat

In foot flat, or loading response phase, the body absorbs the impact of the foot by rolling in pronation. The hip moves slowly into extension, caused by a contraction of the adductor magnus and gluteus maximus muscles. The knee flexes to 15° to 20° of flexion. Ankle plantarflexion increases to 10-15°.

Midstance

In midstance, the hip moves from 10° of flexion to extension by contraction of the gluteus medius muscle. The knee reaches maximal flexion and then begins to extend. The ankle becomes supinated and dorsiflexed (5°), which is caused by some contraction of the triceps surae muscles. During this phase, the body is supported by one single leg. At this moment the body begins to move from force absorption at impact to force propulsion forward.

Heel Off

Heel off begins when the heel leaves the floor. In this phase, the bodyweight is divided over the metatarsal heads.Here can we see 10-13° of hip hyperextension, which then goes into flexion. The knee becomes flexed (0-5°) and the ankle supinates and plantar flexes.

Toe Off

In the toe-off/pre-swing phase, the hip becomes less extended. The knee is flexed 35-40° and plantar flexion of the ankle increases to 20°.In toe-off, like the name says, the toes leave the ground.

Early Swing

In the early swing, phase the hip extends to 10° and then flexes due to contraction of the iliopsoas muscle 20° with lateral rotation. The knee flexes to 40-60°, and the ankle goes from 20° of plantar flexion to dorsiflexion, to end in a neutral position.

Mid Swing

In the midswing, phase the hip flexes to 30° (by contraction of the adductors) and the ankle becomes dorsiflexed due to a contraction of the tibialis anterior muscle.The knee flexes 60° but then extends approximately 30° due to the contraction of the sartorius muscle.This extension is caused by the quadriceps muscles.

Late Swing

The late swing/declaration phase begins with hip flexion of 25-30°, a locked extension of the knee and a neutral position of the ankle.

Anatomical Considerations

The gait cycle involves movement in each part of the leg (and the body).

In the pelvic region, there is an anterior-posterior displacement, which alternates from left to right. This displacement facilitates anterior movement of the leg. At each side, there is an anterior-posterior displacement of 4-5°.

In the frontal plane, varus movement is observed in the foot between heel-strike and foot-flat and between heel-off and toe-off. Some valgus movement is also observed between foot-flat and heel off in the feet. In the hip, some varus movement is observed in lateral movements. When the abductors are too weak, a Trendelenburg gait can be observed.

It is important to recognize that the entire body moves while walking. A disorder in any segment of the body can have consequences on the individual's gait pattern, like a reduced knee flexion range in patients with a reconstructed ACL.

Pathological Gait

Pathological gait is an altered gait pattern due to deformities, weakness or other impairments, for example, loss of motor control or pain. Alterations can broadly be divided into neurological or musculoskeletal causes.

Musculoskeletal Causes

Pathological gait patterns resulting from musculoskeletal are often caused by soft tissue imbalance, joint alignment or bony abnormalities. Infliction of these on one joint often then impacts on other joints, affecting the gait pattern as a result. The common deviation can be categorised broadly as:

- Hip pathology.

- Knee pathology.

- Foot and ankle pathology.

- Leg length discrepancy.

- Pain.

Hip Pathology

Arthritis is a common cause of pathological gait. An arthritic hip has reduced range of movement during swing phase which causes an exaggeration of movement in the opposite limb hip hiking.

Excessive Hip Flexion can significantly alter gait pattern most commonly due to:

- Flexion contractures.

- IT band contractures.

- Hip flexor spasticity.

- Compensation for excessive knee flexion and ankle DF.

- Hip pain.

- Compensation for excess ankle plantar flexion in mid swing.

The deviation of stance phase will occur mainly on the affected side. The result is forward tilt of the trunk and increased demand on the hip extensors or increased lordosis of the spine with anterior pelvic tilt. A person with reduced spinal mobility will adopt a forward flexion position in order to alter their centre of gravity permanently during gait.

Hip Abductor Weakness: The abductor muscles stabilise the pelvis to allow the opposite leg to lift during the swing phase. Weak abductor muscles will cause the hip to drop towards the side of the leg swinging forward. This is also known as Trendelenburg gait.

Hip Adductor Contracture: During swing phase the leg crosses midline due to the weak adductor muscles, this is known as 'scissor gait'.

Weak Hip Extensors will cause a person to take a smaller step to lessen the hip flexion required for initial contact, resulting in a lesser force of contraction required from the extensors. Overall gait will be slower to allow time for limb stabilisation. Compensation is increased posterior trunk positioning to maintain alignment of the pelvis in relation to the trunk.

Hip Flexor Weakness results in a smaller step length due to the weakness of the muscle to create the forward motion. Gait will likely be slower and may result in decreased floor clearance of the toes and create a drag.

Knee Pathologies

Weak Quadriceps: The quadriceps role is to eccentrically control the knee during flexion through the stance phase. If these muscles are weak the hip extensors will compensate by bringing the limb back into a more extended position, reducing the amount of flexion at the knee during stance phase. Alternatively heel strike will occur earlier increasing the ankle of plantar flexion at the ankle, preventing the forward movement of the tibia, to help stabilise the knee joint.

Severe Quadriceps Weakness or instability at the knee joint will present in hyperextension during the initial contact to stance phase. The knee joint will 'snap' back into hyperextension as the bodyweight moves forwards over the limb.

Knee Flexion Contraction will cause a limping type gait pattern. The knee is restricted in extension, meaning heel strike is limited and step length reduced. To compensate the person is likely to 'toe walk' during stance phase. Knee flexion contractures of more than 30 degrees will be obvious during normal paced gait. Contractures less then this will be more evident with increased speeds.

Ankle Pathologies

Ankle Dorsiflexion Weakness results in a lack of heel strike and decreased floor clearance. This leads to an increased step height and prolonged swing phase.

Calf Tightening or Contractures due to a period of immobilisation or trauma will cause reduced heel strike due to restricted dorsiflexion. The compensated gait result will be 'toe walking' on stance phase, reduced step length and excessive knee and hip flexion during swing phase to ensure floor clearance.

Foot Pathologies

Hallux Rigidus results in a lack of dorsiflexion of the great toe. The MPJ uses the windlass effect to raise the arch and stiffen the foot during dorsiflexion of the hallux. This stiffness increases the efficiency of the propulsion portion of the gait cycle. To be efficient in creating stiffness, the hallux should be able to dorsiflex at least 65 degrees.

Leg Length Discrepancy

Leg length discrepancy can be as a result of an asymmetrical pelvic, tibia or femur length or for other reasons such as a scoliosis or contractures. The gait pattern will present as a pelvic dip to the shortened side during stance phase with possible 'toe walking' on that limb. The opposite leg is likely to increase its knee and hip flexion to reduce its length.

Antalgic Gait

Antalgic gait due to knee pain presents with decreased weight bearing on the affected side. The knee remains in flexion and possible toe weight-bearing occurs during stance phase.

Antalgic gait due to ankle pain may present with a reduced stride length and decreased weight bearing on the affected limb. If the problem is pain in the forefoot then toe-off will be avoided and heel weight-bearing used. If the pain is more in the heel, toe weight-bearing is more likely. General ankle pain may result in weight-bearing on the lateral border.

Antalgic gait due to hip pain results in reduced stance phase on that side. The trunk is propelled quickly forwards with the opposite shoulder lifted in an attempt to even the weight distribution over the limb and reduce weight-bearing. Swing phase is also reduced.

Common Neurological Causes of Pathological Gait

Hemiplegic Gait, often seen as a result of a stroke. The upper limb is in a flexed position, adducted and internally rotated at the shoulder. The lower limb is internally rotated, knee extended and the ankle inverted and plantarflexed. The gait is likely to be slow with circumduction or hip hitching of the affected limb to aid floor clearance.

Diplegic Gait: Spasticity is normally associated with both lower limbs. Contractures of the adductor muscles can create a 'scissor' type gait with a narrowed base of support. Spasticity in the lower half of the legs results in plantarflexed ankles presenting in 'tiptoe' walking and often toe dragging. Excessive hip and knee flexion is required to overcome this.

Parkinsonian Gait often seen in Parkinson's disease or associated with conditions that cause parkinsonisms. Rigidity of joints results in reduced arm swing for balance. A stooped posture and flexed knees are a common presentation. Bradykinesia causes small steps that are shuffling in presentation. There may be occurrences of freezing or short rapid bursts of steps known as 'festination' and turning can be difficult.

Ataxic Gait is seen as uncoordinated steps with a wide base of support and staggering/variable foot placement. This gait is associated with cerebellar disturbances and can be seen in patients with longstanding alcohol dependency.

People with 'Sensory' Disturbances may present with a sensory ataxic gait. Presentation is a wide base of support, high steps, and slapping of feet on the floor in order to gain some sensory feedback. They may also need to rely on observation of foot placement and will often look at the floor during mobility due to a lack of proprioception.

Myopathic Gait: Due to hip muscular dystrophy, if it is bilateral the presentation will be a 'waddling gait', unilaterally will present as a Trendelenburg Gait.

Neuropathic Gaits: High stepping gait to gain floor clearance often due to foot drop.

Gait Analysis

The analysis of the gait cycle is important in the biomechanical mobility examination to gain information about lower limb dysfunction in dynamic movement and loading. When analysing the gait cycle, it is best to examine one joint at a time. Objective and subjective methods can be used.

CORE

In common parlance, the core of the body is broadly considered to be the torso. Functional movements are highly dependent on this part of the body, and lack of core muscular development can result in a predisposition to injury. The major muscles of the core reside in the area of the belly and the mid and lower back (not the shoulders), and peripherally include the hips, the shoulders and the neck.

Muscles

Major muscles included are the pelvic floor muscles, transversus abdominis, multifidus, internal and external obliques, rectus abdominis, erector spinae (sacrospinalis) especially the longissimus thoracis, and the diaphragm. The lumbar muscles, quadratus Lumborum (deep portion), deep rotators, as well as cervical muscles, rectus capitus anterior and lateralis, longus coli may also be considered members of the core group.

Minor core muscles include the latissimus dorsi, gluteus maximus, and trapezius.

Functions of the Core

The core is used to stabilize the thorax and the pelvis during dynamic movement and it also provides internal pressure to expel substances (vomit, feces, carbon-laden air, etc.).

- Continence.

Continence is the ability to withhold bowel movements, and urinary stress incontinence (the lack of bladder control due to pelvic floor dysfunction) can result from weak core musculature.

- Pregnancy.

Women use their core muscles, specifically the transversus abdominis, during labor and delivery.

- Valsalva maneuver.

Core muscles are also involved in the Valsalva maneuver, where the thorax tightens while the breath is held to assist, often involuntarily, in activities such as lifting, pushing, excretion and birthing.

Anatomical Posture and Support

The core is traditionally assumed to originate most full-body functional movement, including most sports. In addition, the core determines to a large part a person's posture. In all, the human anatomy is built to take force upon the bones and direct autonomic force, through various joints, in the desired direction. The core muscles align the spine, ribs, and pelvis of a person to resist a specific force, whether static or dynamic.

Static Core Function

Static core functionality is the ability of one's core to align the skeleton to resist a force that does not change.

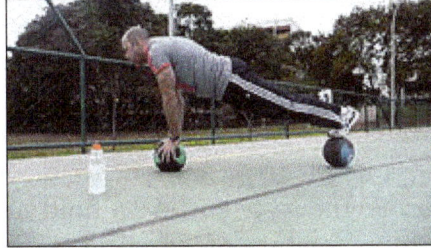

Medicine Ball Plank.

Example of Static Core Function

An example of static core function is firing a rifle in the prone position. To maintain accuracy, the shooter must be able to transfer his or her own body weight and the weight of the rifle into the earth. Any attempt of the shooter to create a dynamic motion of the sights (muscle the sights onto the target vs. allowing the posture to aim) will result in a jerky posture where the sights do not sit still on the target. For the shooter to maintain accuracy, the muscles cannot exert force on the rifle, and the skeleton must be aligned to set the rifle (and therefore the sights) onto the target. The core, while resting on the ground and relatively far away from the rifle, is nevertheless aligning the spine and pelvis to which the shoulder and arms and neck are connected. For these peripheral elements to remain static, and not move unnecessarily, the spine, pelvis, and rib cage must be aligned towards this end. Thus the core muscles provide support of the axial skeleton (skull, spine, and tailbone) in an alignment where the upper body can provide a steady, solid base for the rifle to remain motionless.

- Resistance: Gravity.

- Plane of movement: Coronal (side to side), Sagittal (forward and behind the anatomical position).

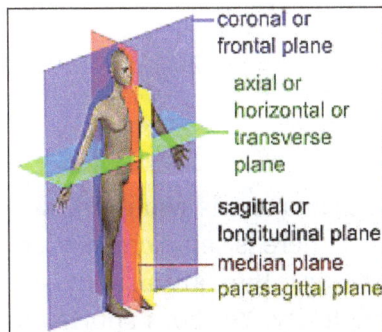

The main anatomical planes of the human body, including median (red), parasagittal (yellow), frontal or coronal plane (blue) and transverse or axial plane (green).

Dynamic Core Function

The nature of dynamic movement must take into account our skeletal structure (as a lever) in addition to the force of external resistance, and consequently incorporates a vastly different complex of muscles and joints versus a static position.

Because of this functional design, during dynamic movement there is more dependence on core musculature than just skeletal rigidity as in a static situation. This is because the purpose of movement is not to resist a static, unchanging resistance, but to resist a force that changes its plane of motion. By incorporating movement, the bones of the body must absorb the resistance in a fluid manner, and thus tendons, ligaments, muscles, and innervation take on different responsibilities. These responsibilities include postural reactions to changes in speed (quickness of a contraction), motion (reaction time of a contraction) and power (amount of resistance resisted in a period of time).

Example of Dynamic Core Function

An example of this is walking on a slope. The body must resist gravity while moving in a direction, and balancing itself on uneven ground. This forces the body to align the bones in a way that balances the body while at the same time achieving momentum through pushing against the ground in the opposite direction of the desired movement. Initially, it may seem that the legs are the prime movers of this action, but without balance, the legs will only cause the person to fall over. Therefore, the prime mover of walking is achieving core stability, and then the legs move this stable core by using the leg muscles.

FUNCTIONAL MOVEMENT

Functional movements are movements based on real-world situational biomechanics. They usually involve multi-planar, multi-joint movements which place demand on the body's core musculature and innervation.

Functional vs. other Movements

Sports-specific

Sports-specific movements, such as a tennis swing or bowling a cricket ball, are based on sports-specific situations. While there is some cross-over application from sports-specific movements (such as running), they are usually so specific that they supersede functional movements in complexity. Yet both sports and functional movements are dependent on the body's core.

Muscle-specific

Traditional weight-lifting depends on muscle-specific program-design with the goal of muscle-specific hypertrophy. For example, a concentration biceps curl attempts to isolate the biceps brachii, although by gripping the weight one also engages the wrist flexors. These exercises tend to be the most far-removed from functional movement, due to their attempt to micromanage the variables acting on the individual muscles. Functional exercises, on the other hand, attempt to incorporate as many variables as possible (balance, multiple joints, multiple planes of movement), thus decreasing the load on the muscle but increasing the complexity of motor coordination and flexibility.

Biomechanics

Functional movement usually involves gross motor movement involving the core, which refers to the muscles of the abdomen and spine, such as segmental stabilizers.

FUNCTIONAL SPINAL UNIT

A functional spinal unit (FSU) (or motion segment) is the smallest physiological motion unit of the spine to exhibit biomechanical characteristics similar to those of the entire spine.

A FSU consists of two adjacent vertebrae, the intervertebral disc and all adjoining ligaments between them and excludes other connecting tissues such as muscles. The three-joint complex that results is sometimes referred to as the "articular triad".

In vitro studies of isolated or multiple, FSU's are often used to measure biomechanical properties of the spine. The typical load-displacement behavior of a cadaveric FSU specimen is nonlinear. Within the total range of passive motion of any FSU, the typical load-displacement curve consists of 2 regions or 'zones' that exhibit very different biomechanical behavior. In the vicinity of the resting neutral position of the FSU, this load-displacement behavior is highly flexible. This is the region known as the 'neutral zone', which is the motion region of the joint where the passive osteoligamentous stability mechanisms exert little or no influence. During passive physiological movement of the FSU, motion occurs in this region against minimal internal resistance. It is a region in which a small load causes a relatively large displacement. The 'elastic zone' is the remaining region of FSU motion that continues from the end of the neutral zone to the point of maximum resistance (provided by the passive osteoligamentous stability mechanism), thus limiting the range of motion.

Mechanome

The mechanome consists of the body, or ome, of data including cell and molecular processes relating to force and mechanical systems at molecular, cellular and tissue length scales - the fundamental "machine code" structures of the cell. The mechanome encompasses biological motors, like kinesin, myosin, RNAP, and Ribosome mechanical structures, like actin or the cytoskeleton and also proteomic and genomic components that are mechanosensitive and are involved in the response of cells to externally applied force.

A definition of the "Mechanome" extending to cell/organ/body given by Prof. Roger Kamm, at the 5th World Congress of Biomechanics Munich, includes understanding: The complete state of stress existing from tissues to cells to molecules. The biological state that results from the distribution of forces. Requires knowledge of the distribution of force throughout the cell/organ/body, the functional interactions between these stresses and the fundamental biological processes.

The mechanome seeks to understand the fundamental physical-mechanical processes and events that affect biological function. An example at the molecular level includes the common structural designs used by kinesin and myosin motor proteins (such as dimer formation and mechanochemical cycles) that control their function and lead to properties such as processivity. The mechanome assembles the common features of these motors regardless of the "track" (microtubules, actin filaments, nucleotide based structures, membranes) they move on. A cytoskeletal example includes structures such as actin filament networks and bundles that can form from a variety of actin binding proteins that cross-link or bundle actin filaments leading to common mechanical changes of these structures. A cell machinery example includes common structures such as contractile ring formation formed by both actin and tubulin type structures leading to the same mechanical result of cell division.

In order to respond to loading cells require a functional mechanome, defined as the cellular and extracellular mechanosensitive elements (genomic, proteomic, metabolic etc.) that contribute to the mechanical responsiveness of specific cells within a defined mechanical environment.

Using mechanical force techniques, such as optical tweezers or atomic force microscopy, single proteins can be identified by a unique structural fingerprint .

Mechanomics

Mechanomics is the study of how forces are transmitted and the influence they have on biological function.

Mechanomics is also an emerging field between biology and biomechanics.

MOVEMENT ASSESSMENT

Movement assessment is the practice of analysing movement performance during functional tasks to determine the kinematics of individual joints and their effect on the kinetic chain. Three-dimensional or two-dimensional analysis of the biomechanics involved in sporting tasks can assist in prevention of injury and enhancing athletic performance. Identification of abnormal movement mechanics provides physical therapists with the ability to prescribe more accurate corrective exercise programs to prevent injury and improve exercise rehabilitation and progression following injury and assist in determining readiness to return to sport.

Landing Error Scoring System (LESS)

The LESS is a valid and reliable tool for the biomechanical assessment of the jump landing technique. The LESS involves the scoring of 22 biomechanical criteria of the lower extremity and trunk, with the outcomes being associated with the risk of anterior cruciate ligament (ACL) and patellofemoral injury. LESS scoring is split into the following categories: excellent (0-3); good (4-5); moderate (6-7); and poor (>7). Identification of biomechanical abnormalities in landing technique, the effect of fatigue and differences between gender allow for more precise clinical exercise intervention to reduce the risk of injury.

Unsupported Single Leg Squat

The single leg squat is an exercise that was developed into a functional test by Liebenson to examine the biomechanics of the lower extremity, assess hip muscle dysfunction and provide an indication of mechanics during daily functional tasks. The test requires the person to stand on the limb being tested, with the non-weight bearing limb in about 45° of hip flexion and about 90° of knee flexion. The person's arms should be in 90° of shoulder flexion and full elbow extension. The athlete is required to squat down to at least 60° of knee flexion and return to the start position within 6 seconds.

Single Leg Hop for Distance

Single leg hop tests are commonly used to assess functional knee performance by assessing limb symmetry after an anterior cruciate ligament injury or following anterior cruciate ligament reconstruction. The hop tests mainly used are: the single leg hop for distance; crossover hop test; triple hop test; 6m timed hop test; square hop test and side-to-side hop test. The limb symmetry is assessed by means of the limb symmetry index (LSI). Normal values for return to play criteria following ACL reconstruction indicate that the injured limb should be greater than or equal to 90% of the uninjured limb.

WOMERSLEY NUMBER

The Womersley number (α or W_0) is a dimensionless number in biofluid mechanics and biofluid dynamics. It is a dimensionless expression of the pulsatile flow frequency in relation to viscous effects. It is named after John R. Womersley (1907–1958) for his work with blood flow in arteries. The Womersley number is important in keeping dynamic similarity when scaling an experiment. An example of this is scaling up the vascular system for experimental study. The Womersley number is also important in determining the thickness of the boundary layer to see if entrance effects can be ignored.

This number is also referred to as Stokes number, S_t, due to the pioneering work done by Sir George Stokes on the Stokes second problem.

Derivation

The Womersley number, usually denoted α, is defined by the relation:

$$\alpha^2 = \frac{\text{transient inertial force}}{\text{viscous force}} = \frac{\rho \omega U}{\mu U L^{-2}} = \frac{\omega L^2}{\mu \rho^{-1}} = \frac{\omega L^2}{\nu},$$

where L is an appropriate length scale (for example the radius of a pipe), ω is the angular frequency of the oscillations, and ν, ρ, μ are the kinematic viscosity, density, and dynamic viscosity of the fluid, respectively. The Womersley number is normally written in the powerless form:

$$\alpha = L \left(\frac{\omega \rho}{\mu} \right)^{\frac{1}{2}}.$$

In the cardiovascular system, the pulsation frequency decreases as the blood is distanced from the origin of pulsation, the heart. However, the Womersley number, like many characteristic numbers, defines a system by order of magnitude (OoM). The pulsation frequency maintains a single OoM throughout the body (<1 s^-1) and is square rooted in the Womersley equation, reducing the OoM further. Therefore, the frequency change in blood flow does not affect the characteristics defined by the Womersley number.

Characteristic length, or in the case of blood flow, the diameter of the vessel, is a defining characteristic of a system and often the driving factor of characteristic numbers. Since the vessel diameters in the body differ up to three OoM, the Womersley number will depend predominantly on diameter. That being said, using standard values for frequency, viscosity and density, the Womersley number of human blood flow can be estimated as follows:

$$\alpha = L \left(\frac{\omega \rho}{\mu} \right)^{\frac{1}{2}}.$$

Below is a list of estimated Womersley numbers in different human blood vessels:

Vessel	Diameter (m)	α
Aorta	0.025	13.83
Artery	0.004	2.21
Arteriole	$3 \cdot 10^{-5}$	0.0166
Capillary	$8 \cdot 10^{-6}$	$4.43 \cdot 10^{-3}$
Venule	$2 \cdot 10{-5}$	0.011
Veins	0.005	2.77
Vena cava	0.03	16.6

It can also be written in terms of the dimensionless Reynolds number (Re) and Strouhal number (St):

$$\alpha = \left(2\pi \mathrm{ReSt}\right)^{1/2}.$$

The Womersley number arises in the solution of the linearized Navier–Stokes equations for oscillatory flow (presumed to be laminar and incompressible) in a tube. It expresses the ratio of the transient or oscillatory inertia force to the shear force. When α is small (1 or less), it means the frequency of pulsations is sufficiently low that a parabolic velocity profile has time to develop during each cycle, and the flow will be very nearly in phase with the pressure gradient, and will be given to a good approximation by Poiseuille's law, using the instantaneous pressure gradient. When α is large (10 or more), it means the frequency of pulsations is sufficiently large that the velocity profile is relatively flat or plug-like, and the mean flow lags the pressure gradient by about 90 degrees. Along with the Reynolds number, the Womersley number governs dynamic similarity.

The boundary layer thickness δ that is associated with the transient acceleration is inversely related to the Womersley number. This can be seen by recognizing the Womersley number as the square root of the Stokes number.

$$\delta = \left(L/\alpha\right) = \left(\frac{L}{\sqrt{\mathrm{Stk}}}\right),$$

where L is a characteristic length.

Biofluid Mechanics

In a flow distribution network that progresses from a large tube to many small tubes (e.g. a blood vessel network), the frequency, density, and dynamic viscosity are (usually) the same throughout the network, but the tube radii change. Therefore, the Womersley number is large in large vessels and small in small vessels. As the vessel diameter decreases with each division the Womersley number soon becomes quite small. The Womersley numbers tend to 1 at the level of the terminal arteries. In the arterioles, capillaries, and venules the Womersley numbers are less than one. In these regions the inertia force becomes less important and the flow is determined by the balance of viscous stresses and the pressure gradient. This is called microcirculation.

Some typical values for the Womersley number in the cardiovascular system for a canine at a heart rate of 2 Hz are:

- Ascending aorta — 13.2.
- Descending aorta — 11.5.
- Abdominal aorta — 8.
- Femoral artery — 3.5.
- Carotid artery — 4.4.
- Arterioles —0.04.
- Capillaries — 0.005.
- Venules — 0.035.
- Inferior vena cava — 8.8.
- Main pulmonary artery — 15.

It has been argued that universal biological scaling laws (power-law relationships that describe variation of quantities such as metabolic rate, lifespan, length, etc., with body mass) are a consequence of the need for energy minimization, the fractal nature of vascular networks, and the crossover from high to low Womersley number flow as one progresses from large to small vessels.

TINETTI TEST

The Tinetti-test was published by Mary Tinetti (Yale University) to assess the gait and balance in older adults and to assess perception of balance and stability during activities of daily living and fear of falling. It is also called Performance-Oriented Mobility Assessment (POMA). It also is a very good indicator of the fall risk of an individual. It has better test-retest, discriminative and predictive validities concerning fall risk than other tests including Timed Up and Go test (TUG), one-leg stand and functional reach test.

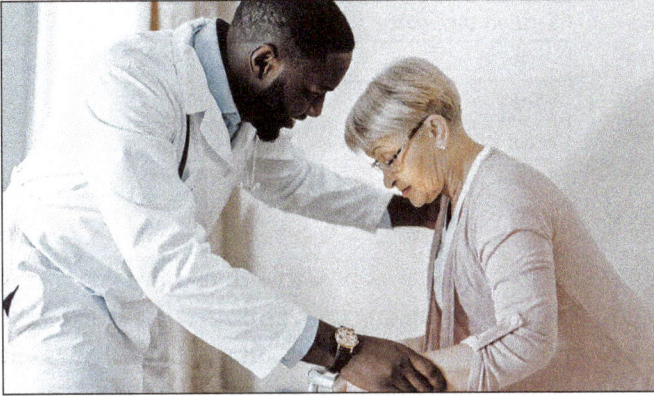

Intended Population

It is used in various settings eg. those diagnosed with Multiple Sclerosis, Parkinson's Disease, acquired brain injury, spinal cord injury, stroke and the elderly population.

Procedure

The test requires a hard armless chair, a stopwatch and also, a 15 feet even and uniform walkway. It has 2 sections: one assesses balance abilities in a chair and also in standing; the other assesses dynamic balance during gait on a 15 feet even walkway.

The patient is to sit in an armless chair and will be asked to rise up and stay standing. The patient will then turn 360° and then sit back down. This is to test the patients' balance. Testing this, the evaluator will look at several key points including how does the patient rise from and sits down on his/her chair, whether or not the patient stays upright while sitting and standing, what happens when the patients' eyes are closed or when the patient gets a small push against the sternum.

Next, the patient will have to walk a few meters at a normal speed, followed by turning and walking back at a "fast but safe" speed. The patient will then sit back down. As well as in the first part of the test, there are some points the evaluator has to look at. These are the length and height of the steps, the symmetry and continuity of the steps and straightness of the trunk.

During this test, the patient can use any assistive devices (walking stick, crutches, zimmer frame) they would normally use.

Interpretation

The Tinetti test has a gait score and a balance score. It uses a 3-point ordinal scale of 0, 1 and 2. Gait is scored over 12 and balance is scored over 16 totalling 28. The lower the score on the Tinetti test, the higher the risk of falling.

Tinneti tool score	Risk of fall
≤ 18	High
19-23	Moderate
≥ 24	Low

Gait and Balance

If the patient needs to rise in stages, it is possible that there is a problem with proprioception or cerebellar problems. A shuffling gait, abnormal knee extension, high stepping, toe dragging and an inability to stop or turn are all signs of abnormalities during walking. These signs need to be further evaluated because they could indicate several health problems such as partial vision loss, lowered strength in the knee or hip joints, problems with proprioception, frontal lobe dysfunction or even vascular claudication. When the patient falls into his/her chair upon returning it is indicative of poor knee and/or hip flexion.

Clinimetric Properties

The test and retest values for the POMA-T, POMA-B en POMA-G all varied between .72 and .86. The interrater reliability values all varied between .80 and .93.6 People with a score lower than 26 will have a higher chance of falling. This test has a sensitivity of 70% and a specificity of 52%. This means that 70% of the people with a higher fall risk will have a test score lower than 26. It also means that 52% of the people who have a test score lower than 26 have a higher fall risk and will have a fall within a year. The people who have a score of 26 or lower have a two-fold risk of falling.

References

- Balance: physio-pedia.com, Retrieved 13 July, 2019

- Nichols, W. W., O'Rourke, M. F. (2005). McDonald's Blood Flow in Arteries (5th ed.). London (England): Hodder-Arnold. ISBN 978-0-340-80941-9

- Base-of-Support: physio-pedia.com, Retrieved 17 August, 2019

- Gribble, P.A.; Hertek, J. (2004). "Effect of Lower-Extremity Fatigue on Postural Control". Archives of Physical Medicine and Rehabilitation. 85 (4): 589–592. doi:10.1016/j.apmr.2003.06.031. PMID 15083434

- Ground-reaction-force-grf: kistler.com, Retrieved 09 July, 2019

- Juras, Grzegorz; Słomka, Kajetan; Fredyk, Artur; Sobota, Grzegorz; Bacik, Bogdan (2008). "Evaluation of the Limits of Stability (LOS) Balance Test". Journal of Human Kinetics. 19: 39–52 doi:10.2478/v10078-008-0003-0

4

Tissue Biomechanics

Tissue biomechanics deals with the study of functions of bone, tendons and muscles to an external force. The mechanical causes of damage on these tissues are also studied within this field. This chapter has been carefully written to provide an easy understanding of tissue biomechanics.

The mechanics of soft or hard biological tissues is a multidisciplinary topic and rapidly expanding research area from different scientific areas, including biology, medicine, physics, materials science, mechanics, applied mathematics and computational physics. The word "Biomechanics" means mechanics applied to biology. Mechanics and living tissues and structures are often opposed: the first is rigid and repetitive, while the second is flexible and capable of improvisation. It thus seems paradoxical to want to explain mechanically biological phenomena and thus reduce the living to a simple human production, as the project of biology and mechanism wants. The mechanical model was nevertheless considered sufficient to describe biological structures by the French philosopher Descartes at the macroscopic level; at the microscopic level, biologists speak of "physico-chemical mechanisms". The analogy is reinforced by the etymology of the word "organ", which comes from "tool", and the organs are then natural tools. Even if this is only an analogy, living beings can thus be considered as technical objects; we are technically capable of treating living beings as machines, producing tissues or organs of substitution. In this mechanistic and deterministic perspective, it is the organ that creates the function, not the reverse, from a finalist point of view. Descartes in his time already compares the human body to a machine (automaton) to make medicine a science: the heart is assimilated to a pump, its two cavities to locks, veins to streams, nerves to nets, the joints to pulleys. The analogy is less structural than functional: it does not pretend to explain the nature of organs, but their functions, by identifying the causes of their movements.

The general purpose of mechanics for living organisms is to explore the mechanical properties of living organisms and to analyze the principles of engineering that make biological systems work. It deals with the existing relationships between structures and functions at all levels of life organization, from the molecular level (collagen, elastin) to tissues and organs. It can be divided into several sub-disciplines, each with its own field of investigation: biomechanics characterizes the spatio-temporal responses of biological materials – solid, fluid or viscoelastic – to internal and external constraints.

The coinagemechanobiology has been invented to highlight the fact that a number of biological processes at different scales are sensitive to local mechanical fields. In addition to classical mechanics, biomechanics uses various disciplines and techniques such as rheology (study of the behavior of biological fluids such as blood) and resistance of materials to model stresses undergone by living tissues (e.g. cartilage of the joints, bones) and solid mechanics to analyze motricity and locomotion, from individual cells to whole organisms.

In this exploration of living structures, whose specifications are demanding (variability of properties, heterogeneity, multiscale and multiphysical behaviors, structural and behavioral complexity must all ideally be considered), mechanics has already developed a wide range of themes and methods, amongst which we can cite: the strength of materials, hydraulics, elasticity, but also the mechanics of heterogeneous and anisotropic continuous media, soft or hard, the mechanics of multiphase deformable porous media, involving coupled phenomena including chemical reactions, transport and mass transfer, as well as electrical interactions due to the presence of charged ions and macromolecules.

Although the origin of Biomechanics can be traced back to Aristotle, the field of Biomechanics has expanded in a tremendous manner since the early 1980s and advances have been made on many fronts. The necessarily multidisciplinary approach and the multiscale aspects of living tissues make it difficult to apprehend all aspects of their mechanical response, starting from the cellular level up to the tissue level. Biology includes a lot of descriptive material and understanding the cellular mechanisms responsible for the tissue mechanical response at the macroscale as well as their time evolution due to growth and remodeling remains very challenging for non-biologists. On the other hand, mechanics is more quantitative in nature and requires some mathematical knowledge which is not easily understandable for researchers in medicine, biology or even materials science.

The classical framework of continuum mechanics which holds for continuous bodies with a constant mass has clearly to be enlarged to be able to treat and model biological phenomena under the umbrella of a field theory which treats all variables as continuous (fields) in space and time. Especially, the mechanical modeling of living tissues raises several challenges due to the following novel aspects to be considered in comparison to non-living materials and structures:

- Biological tissues are prone to a biological evolution due to growth or remodeling phenomena, so that addition of mass due to transport of nutrients, modification of density and properties, shape and topology modifications of the tissue microstructure shave ideally to be accounted for as new phenomena. This requires the reformulation of classical approaches (which were developed for inert materials) for the mechanics of continuous media, in order to take into account their adaptability to their environment. Moreover, one has to expand the thermodynamics of irreversible processes to account for a mass source and flux within the growing domain and to adopt the thermodynamics of open systems as a more natural framework.

- The microstructural evolution of biological tissues involves simultaneous genetic and epigenetic factors, including stress and strains, so that they adapt to mechanical signals and respond by changing their topology, shape, and mechanical properties. The functional adaptation of living tissues has raised a lot of work in the literature, and still remains challenging for researchers in mechanics.

- Since the time evolution of biological tissues occurs at the cellular level, cellular phenomena ideally have to be incorporated into any modeling. Despite the many approaches to account for mechanotransduction, a clear view of the mechanisms though which cells feel signals from their environment and react to them is still not available.

- Notwithstanding biological aspects, the mechanical response of living tissues involves mechanisms at different scales, so a multiscale integrated approach is needed so that the mechanical response at one scale is transferred to the next scale.

- Since biological tissues experience interactions between transport phenomena, chemical reactions and generation of internal stresses, a multiphysical approach is further needed.

- The growth of living tissues involves the addition of new particles to the initial domain, which would require considering a change of the domain topology, which is not accounted for in the classical framework of continuum mechanics.

- From the point of view of measurements, the methods of investigation of living tissues require the probing of objects with heterogeneous characteristics, structurally complex and variable in terms of behavior. The characterization is done in vitro and in vivo and tries to take into account the variability and the uncertainty of the response. In addition to conventional mechanical tests (tensile compression, waves, ultrasound, etc.) and field measurements, new techniques have emerged, such as nanomechanics, microfluidics, acoustics, PIV and picoseconds. The following imaging methods are widely used: optical, NMR, MRI, SEM, ultrasound, confocal microscopy, X-ray microscopy, tomography, elastography and Raman spectroscopy.

HARD TISSUE

Hard tissue (also termed calcified tissue) is tissue which is mineralized and has a firm intercellular matrix. The hard tissues of humans are bone, tooth enamel, dentin, and cementum. The term is in contrast to soft tissue.

Enamel

Enamel is the hardest substance in the human body and contains the highest percentage of minerals, 96%, with water and organic material composing the rest. The primary mineral is hydroxyapatite, which is a crystalline calcium phosphate. Enamel is formed on the tooth while the tooth is developing within the gum, before it erupts into the mouth. Once fully formed, it does not contain blood vessels or nerves. Remineralisation of teeth can repair damage to the tooth to a certain degree but damage beyond that cannot be repaired by the body. The maintenance and repair of human tooth enamel is one of the primary concerns of dentistry.

In humans, enamel varies in thickness over the surface of the tooth, often thickest at the cusp, up to 2.5 mm, and thinnest at its border with the cementum at the cementoenamel junction (CEJ).

The normal color of enamel varies from light yellow to grayish (bluish) white. At the edges of teeth where there is no dentin underlying the enamel, the color sometimes has a slightly blue tone. Since enamel is semitranslucent, the color of dentin and any material underneath the enamel strongly affects the appearance of a tooth. The enamel on primary teeth has a more opaque crystalline form and thus appears whiter than on permanent teeth.

The large amount of mineral in enamel accounts not only for its strength but also for its brittleness. Tooth enamel ranks 5 on Mohs hardness scale and has a Young's modulus of 83 GPa. Dentin, less mineralized and less brittle, 3–4 in hardness, compensates for enamel and is necessary as a support. On radiographs, the differences in the mineralization of different portions of the tooth and surrounding periodontium can be noted; enamel appears lighter than dentin or pulp since it is denser than both and more radiopaque.

Enamel does not contain collagen, as found in other hard tissues such as dentin and bone, but it does contain two unique classes of proteins: amelogenins and enamelins. While the role of these proteins is not fully understood, it is believed that they aid in the development of enamel by serving as a framework for minerals to form on, among other functions. Once it is mature, enamel is almost totally without the softer organic matter. Enamel is avascular and has no nerve supply within it and is not renewed, however, it is not a static tissue as it can undergo mineralization changes.

Dentin

By weight, 70% of dentin consists of the mineral hydroxylapatite, 20% is organic material, and 10% is water. Yellow in appearance, it greatly affects the color of a tooth due to the translucency of enamel. Dentin, which is less mineralized and less brittle than enamel, is necessary for the support of enamel. Dentin rates approximately 3 on the Mohs scale of mineral hardness.

Cementum

Cementum is slightly softer than dentin and consists of about 45% to 50% inorganic material (hydroxylapatite) by weight and 50% to 55% organic matter and water by weight. The organic portion is composed primarily of collagen and proteoglycans. Cementum is avascular, receiving its nutrition through its own imbedded cells from the surrounding vascular periodontal ligament.

The cementum is light yellow and slightly lighter in color than dentin. It has the highest fluoride content of all mineralized tissue. Cementum also is permeable to a variety of materials. It is formed continuously throughout life because a new layer of cementum is deposited to keep the attachment intact as the superficial layer of cementum ages. Cementum on the root ends surrounds the apical foramen and may extend slightly onto the inner wall of the pulp canal.

SOFT TISSUE

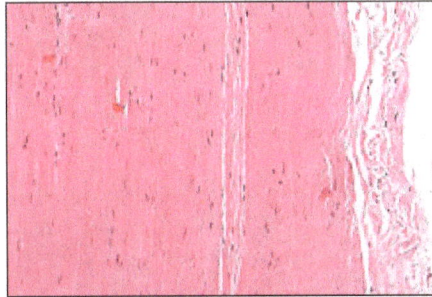

Micrograph of a piece of soft tissue (tendon). H&E stain.

In anatomy, soft tissue includes the tissues that connect, support, or surround other structures and organs of the body, not being hard tissue such as bone. Soft tissue includes tendons, ligaments, fascia, skin, fibrous tissues, fat, and synovial membranes (which are connective tissue), and muscles, nerves and blood vessels (which are not connective tissue).

It is sometimes defined by what it is not. Soft tissue has been defined as "nonepithelial, extraskeletal mesenchyme exclusive of the reticuloendothelial system and glia".

Composition

The characteristic substances inside the extracellular matrix of this kind of tissue are the collagen, elastin and ground substance. Normally the soft tissue is very hydrated because of the ground substance. The fibroblasts are the most common cell responsible for the production of soft tissues' fibers and ground substance. Variations of fibroblasts, like chondroblasts, may also produce these substances.

Mechanical Characteristics

At small strains, elastin confers stiffness to the tissue and stores most of the strain energy. The collagen fibers are comparatively inextensible and are usually loose (wavy, crimped). With increasing tissue deformation the collagen is gradually stretched in the direction of deformation. When taut, these fibers produce a strong growth in tissue stiffness. The composite behavior is analogous to a nylon stocking, whose rubber band does the role of elastin as the nylon does the role of collagen. In soft tissues, the collagen limits the deformation and protects the tissues from injury.

Human soft tissue is highly deformable, and its mechanical properties vary significantly from one person to another. Impact testing results showed that the stiffness and the damping resistance of a test subject's tissue are correlated with the mass, velocity, and size of the striking object. Such properties may be useful for forensics investigation when contusions were induced. When a solid object impacts a human soft tissue, the energy of the impact will be absorbed by the tissues to reduce the effect of the impact or the pain level; subjects with more soft tissue thickness tended to absorb the impacts with less aversion.

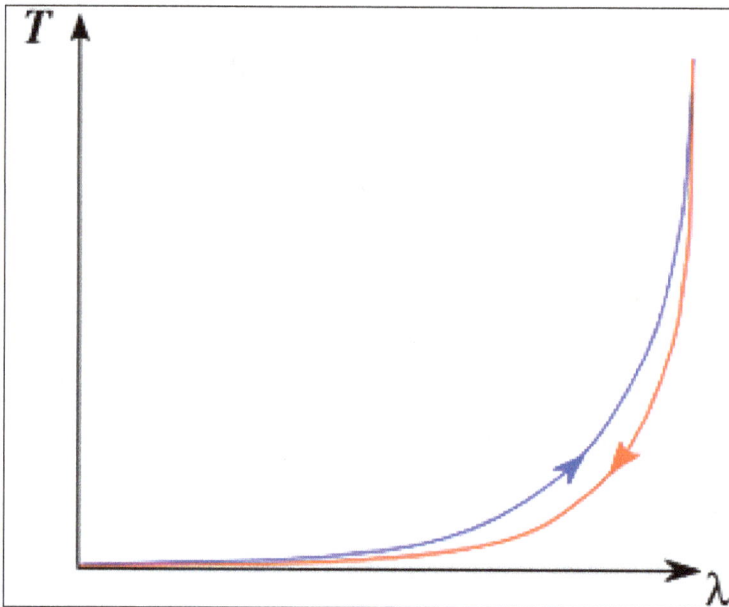

Graph of lagrangian stress (T) versus stretch ratio (λ) of a preconditioned soft tissue.

Soft tissues have the potential to undergo large deformations and still return to the initial configuration when unloaded, i.e. they are hyperelastic materials, and their stress-strain curve is nonlinear. The soft tissues are also viscoelastic, incompressible and usually anisotropic. Some viscoelastic properties observable in soft tissues are: relaxation, creep and hysteresis. In order to describe the mechanical response of soft tissues, several methods have been used. These methods include: hyperelastic macroscopic models based on strain energy, mathematical fits where nonlinear constitutive equations are used, and structurally based models where the response of a linear elastic material is modified by its geometric characteristics.

Pseudoelasticity

Even though soft tissues have viscoelastic properties, i.e. stress as function of strain rate, it can be approximated by a hyperelastic model after precondition to a load pattern. After some cycles of loading and unloading the material, the mechanical response becomes independent of strain rate.

$$\mathbf{S} = \mathbf{S}(\mathbf{E}, \dot{\mathbf{E}}) \quad \rightarrow \quad \mathbf{S} = \mathbf{S}(\mathbf{E})$$

Despite the independence of strain rate, preconditioned soft tissues still present hysteresis, so the mechanical response can be modeled as hyperelastic with different material constants at loading and unloading. By this method the elasticity theory is used to model an inelastic material. Fung has called this model as pseudoelastic to point out that the material is not truly elastic.

Residual Stress

In physiological state, soft tissues usually present residual stress that may be released when the tissue is excised. Physiologists and histologists must be aware of this fact to avoid mistakes when analyzing excised tissues. This retraction usually causes a visual artifact.

Fung-elastic Material

Fung developed a constitutive equation for preconditioned soft tissues which is:

$$W = \frac{1}{2}\left[q + c\left(e^{Q} - 1\right)\right]$$

with,

$$q = a_{ijkl}E_{ij}E_{kl} \qquad Q = b_{ijkl}E_{ij}E_{kl}$$

quadratic forms of Green-Lagrange strains E_{ij} and a_{ijkl}, b_{ijkl} and c material constants. W is the strain energy function per volume unit, which is the mechanical strain energy for a given temperature.

Isotropic Simplification

The Fung-model, simplified with isotropic hypothesis (same mechanical properties in all directions). This written in respect of the principal stretches (λ_i):

$$W = \frac{1}{2}\left[a(\lambda_1^2 + \lambda_2^2 + \lambda_3^2 - 3) + b\left(e^{c(\lambda_1^2 + \lambda_2^2 + \lambda_3^2 - 3)} - 1\right)\right]$$

where a, b and c are constants.

Simplification for Small and Big Stretches

For small strains, the exponential term is very small, thus negligible.

$$W = \frac{1}{2} a_{ijkl} E_{ij} E_{kl}$$

On the other hand, the linear term is negligible when the analysis rely only on big strains.

$$W = \frac{1}{2} c \left(e^{b_{ijkl} E_{ij} E_{kl}} - 1 \right)$$

Gent-elastic Material

$$W = -\frac{\mu J_m}{2} \ln\left(1 - \left(\frac{\lambda_1^2 + \lambda_2^2 + \lambda_3^2 - 3}{J_m}\right)\right)$$

where $\mu > 0$ is the shear modulus for infinitesimal strains and $J_m > 0$ is a stiffening parameter, associated with limiting chain extensibility. This constitutive model cannot be stretched in uni-axial tension beyond a maximal stretch J_m, which is the positive root of:

$$\lambda_m^2 + 2\lambda_m - J_m - 3 = 0$$

Remodeling and Growth

Soft tissues have the potential to grow and remodel reacting to chemical and mechanical long term changes. The rate the fibroblasts produce tropocollagen is proportional to these stimuli. Diseases, injuries and changes in the level of mechanical load may induce remodeling. An example of this phenomenon is the thickening of farmer's hands. The remodeling of connective tissues is well known in bones by the Wolff's law (bone remodeling). Mechanobiology is the science that study the relation between stress and growth at cellular level.

Growth and remodeling have a major role in the cause of some common soft tissue diseases, like arterial stenosis and aneurisms and any soft tissue fibrosis. Other instance of tissue remodeling is the thickening of the cardiac muscle in response to the growth of blood pressure detected by the arterial wall.

Imaging Techniques

There are certain issues that have to be kept in mind when choosing an imaging technique for visualizing soft tissue ECM components. The accuracy of the image analysis relies on the properties and the quality of the raw data and, therefore, the choice of the imaging technique must be based upon issues.

- Having an optimal resolution for the components of interest.

- Achieving high contrast of those components.

- Keeping the artifact count low.

- Having the option of volume data acquisition.

- Keeping the data volume low.

- Establishing an easy and reproducible setup for tissue analysis.

The collagen fibers are approximately 1-2 μm thick. Thus, the resolution of the imaging technique needs to be approximately 0.5 μm. Some techniques allow the direct acquisition of volume data while other need the slicing of the specimen. In both cases, the volume that is extracted must be able to follow the fiber bundles across the volume. High contrast makes segmentation easier, especially when color information is available. In addition, the need for fixation must also be addressed. It has been shown that soft tissue fixation in formalin causes shrinkage, altering the structure of the original tissue. Some typical values of contraction for different fixation are: formalin (5% - 10%), alcohol (10%), bouin (<5%).

Imaging methods used in ECM visualization and their properties.

	Transmission Light	Confocal	Multi-Photon Excitation Fluorescence	Second Harmonic Generation	Optical Coherence Tomography
Resolution	0.25 μm	Axial: 0.25-0.5 μm Lateral: 1 μm	Axial: 0.5 μm Lateral: 1 μm	Axial: 0.5 μm Lateral: 1 μm	Axial: 3-15 μm Lateral: 1-15 μm
Contrast	Very High	Low	High	High	Moderate
Penetration	N/A	10 μm-300 μm	100-1000 μm	100-1000 μm	Up to 2–3 mm
Image stack cost	High	Low	Low	Low	Low
Fixation	Required	Required	Not required	Not required	Not required
Embedding	Required	Required	Not required	Not required	Not required
Staining	Required	Not required	Not required	Not required	Not required
Cost	Low	Moderate to high	High	High	Moderate

BONE

Bone is rigid body tissue consisting of cells embedded in an abundant hard intercellular material. The two principal components of this material, collagen and calcium phosphate, distinguish bone from such other hard tissues as chitin, enamel, and shell. Bone tissue makes up the individual bones of the human skeletal system and the skeletons of other vertebrates.

The functions of bone include (1) structural support for the mechanical action of soft tissues, such as the contraction of muscles and the expansion of lungs, (2) protection of soft organs and tissues, as by the skull, (3) provision of a protective site for specialized tissues such as the blood-forming system (bone marrow), and (4) a mineral reservoir, whereby the endocrine system regulates the level of calcium and phosphate in the circulating body fluids.

Bone is found only in vertebrates, and, among modern vertebrates, it is found only in bony fish and higher classes. Although ancestors of the cyclostomes and elasmobranchs had armoured headcases, which served largely a protective function and appear to have been true bone, modern cyclostomes have only an endoskeleton, or inner skeleton, of noncalcified cartilage and elasmobranchs a skeleton of calcified cartilage. Although a rigid endoskeleton performs obvious body supportive functions for land-living vertebrates, it is doubtful that bone offered any such mechanical advantage to the teleost (bony fish) in which it first appeared, for in a supporting aquatic environment great structural rigidity is not essential for maintaining body configuration. The sharks and rays are superb examples of mechanical engineering efficiency, and their perseverance from the Devonian Period attests to the suitability of their nonbony endoskeleton.

In modern vertebrates, true bone is found only in animals capable of controlling the osmotic and ionic composition of their internal fluid environment. Marine invertebrates exhibit interstitial fluid compositions essentially the same as that of the surrounding seawater. Early signs of regulability are seen in cyclostomes and elasmobranchs, but only at or above the level of true bone fishes does the composition of the internal body fluids become constant. The mechanisms involved in this regulation are numerous and complex and include both the kidney and the gills. Fresh and marine waters provide abundant calcium but only traces of phosphate; because relatively high levels of phosphate are characteristic of the body fluids of higher vertebrates, it seems likely that a large, readily available internal phosphate reservoir would confer significant independence of external environment on bony vertebrates. With the emergence of terrestrial forms, the availability of calcium regulation became equally significant. Along with the kidney and the various component glands of the endocrine system, bone has contributed to development of internal fluid homeostasis—the maintenance of a constant chemical composition. This was a necessary step for the emergence of terrestrial vertebrates. Furthermore, out of the buoyancy of water, structural rigidity of bone afforded mechanical advantages that are the most obvious features of the modern vertebrate skeleton.

Chemical Composition and Physical Properties

Depending upon species, age, and type of bone, bone cells represent up to 15 percent of the volume of bone; in mature bone in most higher animals, they usually represent only up to 5 percent. The nonliving intercellular material of bone consists of an organic component called collagen (a fibrous protein arranged in long strands or bundles similar in structure and organization to the collagen of ligaments, tendons, and skin), with small amounts of proteinpolysaccharides, glycoaminoglycans (formerly known as mucopolysaccharides) chemically bound to protein and dispersed within and around the collagen fibre bundles, and an inorganic mineral component in the form of rod-shaped crystals. These crystals are arranged parallel with the long axes of collagen bundles and many actually lie in voids within the bundles themselves. Organic material constitutes 50 percent of the volume and 30 percent of the dry weight of the intercellular composite, with minerals making up the remainder. The major minerals of the intercellular composite are calcium and phosphate. When first deposited, mineral is crystallographically amorphous, but with maturation it becomes typical of the apatite minerals, the major component being hydroxyapatite. Carbonate is also present—in amounts varying from 4 percent of bone ash in fish and 8 percent in most mammals to more than 13 percent in the turtle—and occurs in two distinct phases, calcium carbonate and a carbonate apatite. Except for that associated with its cellular elements, there is little free water in adult mammalian bone (approximately 8 percent of total volume). As a result, diffusion from surfaces into the interior of the intercellular substance occurs at the slow rates more typical of diffusion from surfaces of solids than within liquids.

The mineral crystals are responsible for hardness, rigidity, and the great compressive strength of bone, but they share with other crystalline materials a great weakness in tension, arising from the tendency for stress to concentrate about defects and for these defects to propagate. On the other hand, the collagen fibrils of bone possess high elasticity, little compressive strength, and considerable intrinsic tensile strength. The tensile strength of bone depends, however, not on collagen alone but on the intimate association of mineral with collagen, which confers on bone many of the general properties exhibited by two-phase materials such as fibre glass and bamboo. In such materials the dispersion of a rigid but brittle material in a matrix of quite different elasticity prevents the propagation of stress failure through the brittle material and therefore allows a closer approach to the theoretical limiting strength of single crystals.

The fine structure of bone has thus far frustrated attempts to determine the true strength of the mineral-matrix composite at the "unit" structural level. Compact (cortical) bone specimens have been found to have tensile strength in the range of 700–1,400 kg per square cm (10,000–20,000 pounds per square inch) and compressive strengths in the range of 1,400–2,100 kg per square cm (20,000–30,000 pounds per square inch). These values are of the same general order as for aluminum or mild steel, but bone has an advantage over such materials in that it is considerably lighter. The great strength of bone exists principally along its long axis and is roughly parallel both to the collagen fibre axis and to the long axis of the mineral crystals.

Although apparently stiff, bones exhibit a considerable degree of elasticity, which is important to the skeleton's ability to withstand impact. Estimates of modulus of elasticity of bone samples are of the order of 420 to 700 kg per square cm (6,000 to 10,000 pounds per square inch), a value much less than steel, for example, indicating the much greater elasticity of bone. Perfect elasticity exists with loads up to 30 to 40 percent of breaking strength; above this, "creep," or gradual deformation, occurs, presumably along natural defects within the bony structure. The modulus of elasticity in bone is strikingly dependent upon the rate at which loads are applied, bones being stiffer during rapid deformation than during slow; this behaviour suggests an element of viscous flow during deformation.

As might be anticipated from consideration of the two-phase composition of bone, variation in the mineral-collagen ratio leads to changes in physical properties: less mineral tends ultimately to greater flexibility and more mineral to increased brittleness. Optimal ratios, as reflected in maximal tensile strength, are observed at an ash content of approximately 66 percent, a value that is characteristic of the weight-bearing bones of mammals.

Bone Morphology

Grossly, bone tissue is organized into a variety of shapes and configurations adapted to the function of each bone: broad, flat plates, such as the scapula, serve as anchors for large muscle masses, while hollow, thick-walled tubes, such as the femur, the radius, and the ulna, support weight or serve as a lever arm. These different types of bone are distinguished more by their external shape than by their basic structure.

All bones have an exterior layer called cortex that is smooth, compact, continuous, and of varying thickness. In its interior, bony tissue is arranged in a network of intersecting plates and spicules called trabeculae, which vary in amount in different bones and enclose spaces filled with blood vessels and marrow. This honeycombed bone is termed cancellous or trabecular. In mature bone, trabeculae are arranged in an orderly pattern that provides continuous units of bony tissue aligned parallel with the lines of major compressive or tensile force. Trabeculae thus provide a complex series of cross-braced interior struts arranged so as to provide maximal rigidity with minimal material.

The central tubular region of the bone, called the diaphysis, flares outward near the end to form the metaphysis, which contains a largely cancellous, or spongy, interior. At the end of the bone is the epiphysis, which in young people is separated from the metaphysis by the physis, or growth plate. The periosteum is a connective sheath covering the outer surface of the bone. The Haversian system, consisting of inorganic substances arranged in concentric rings around the Haversian canals, provides compact bone with structural support and allows for metabolism of bone cells. Osteocytes (mature bone cells) are found in tiny cavities between the concentric rings. The canals contain capillaries that bring in oxygen and nutrients and remove wastes. Transverse branches are known as Volkmann canals.

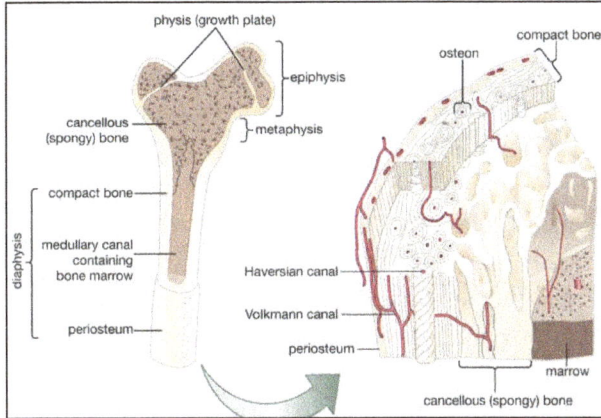

Internal structure of a human long bone, with a magnified cross section of the interior.

Bones such as vertebrae, subject to primarily compressive or tensile forces, usually have thin cortices and provide necessary structural rigidity through trabeculae, whereas bones such as the femur, subject to prominent bending, shear, or torsional forces, usually have thick cortices, a tubular configuration, and a continuous cavity running through their centres (medullary cavity).

Long bones, distinctive of the body's extremities, exhibit a number of common gross structural features. The central region of the bone (diaphysis) is the most clearly tubular. At one or commonly both ends, the diaphysis flares outward and assumes a predominantly cancellous internal structure. This region (metaphysis) functions to transfer loads from weight-bearing joint surfaces to the diaphysis. Finally, at the end of a long bone is a region known as an epiphysis, which exhibits a cancellous internal structure and comprises the bony substructure of the joint surface. Prior to full skeletal maturity the epiphysis is separated from the metaphysis by a cartilaginous plate called the growth plate or physis; in bones with complex articulations (such as the humerus at its lower end) or bones with multiple protuberances (such as the femur at its upper end) there may be several separate epiphyses, each with its growth plate.

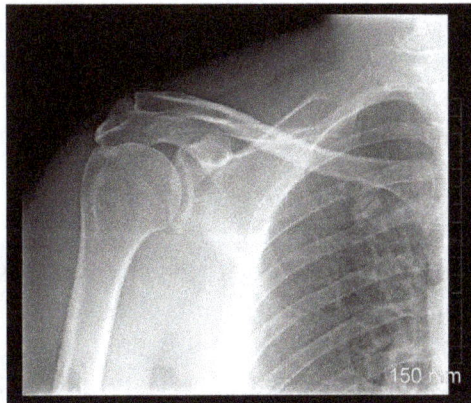

Epiphysis.
Shoulder X-ray showing the epiphysis of the humerus bone in a human.

Four Types of Cells in Bone

Microscopically, bone consists of hard, apparently homogeneous intercellular materi-al, within or upon which can be found four characteristic cell types: osteoblasts, osteo-cytes, osteoclasts, and undifferentiated bone mesenchymal stem cells. Osteoblasts are responsible for the synthesis and deposition on bone surfaces of the protein matrix of new intercellular material. Osteocytes are osteoblasts that have been trapped within in-tercellular material, residing in a cavity (lacuna) and communicating with other osteo-cytes as well as with free bone surfaces by means of extensive filamentous protoplasmic extensions that occupy long, meandering channels (canaliculi) through the bone sub-stance. With the exception of certain higher orders of modern fish, all bone, including primitive vertebrate fossil bone, exhibits an osteocytic structure. Osteoclasts are usu-ally large multinucleated cells that, working from bone surfaces, resorb bone by direct chemical and enzymatic attack. Undifferentiated mesenchymal stem cells of the bone reside in the loose connective tissue between trabeculae, along vascular channels, and in the condensed fibrous tissue covering the outside of the bone (periosteum); they give rise under appropriate stimuli to osteoblasts.

Depending on how the protein fibrils and osteocytes of bone are arranged, bone is of two major types: woven, in which collagen bundles and the long axes of the osteocytes are randomly oriented, and lamellar, in which both the fibrils and osteocytes are aligned in clear layers. In lamellar bone the layers alternate every few micrometres (millionths of a metre), and the primary direction of the fibrils shifts approximately 90°. In com-pact, or cortical, bone of many mammalian species, lamellar bone is further organized into units known as osteons, which consist of concentric cylindrical lamellar elements several millimetres long and 0.2–0.3 mm (0.008–0.012 inch) in diameter. These cyl-inders comprise the haversian systems. Osteons exhibit a gently spiral course oriented along the axis of the bone. In their centre is a canal (haversian canal) containing one or more small blood vessels, and at their outer margins is a boundary layer known as a "cement line," which serves both as a means of fixation for new bone deposited on an old surface and as a diffusion barrier. Osteocytic processes do not penetrate the cement line, and therefore these barriers constitute the outer envelope of a nutritional unit; osteocytes on opposite sides of a cement line derive their nutrition from different vas-cular channels. Cement lines are found in all types of bone, as well as in osteons, and in general they indicate lines at which new bone was deposited on an old surface.

Vascular Supply and Circulation

In a typical long bone, blood is supplied by three separate systems: a nutrient artery, periosteal vessels, and epiphyseal vessels. The diaphysis and metaphysis are nourished primarily by the nutrient artery, which passes through the cortex into the medullary cavity and then ramifies outward through haversian and Volkmann canals to supply the cortex. Extensive vessels in the periosteum, the membrane surrounding the bone, supply the superficial layers of the cortex and connect with the nutrient-artery system.

In the event of obstruction of the nutrient artery, periosteal vessels are capable of meeting the needs of both systems. The epiphyses are supplied by a separate system that consists of a ring of arteries entering the bone along a circular band between the growth plate and the joint capsule. In the adult these vessels become connected to the other two systems at the metaphyseal-epiphyseal junction, but while the growth plate is open there is no such connection, and the epiphyseal vessels are the sole source of nutrition for the growing cartilage; therefore they are essential for skeletal growth.

Drainage of blood is by a system of veins that runs parallel with the arterial supply and by veins leaving the cortical periosteum through muscle insertions. Muscle contraction milks blood outward, giving rise to a centrifugal pattern of flow from the axial nutrient artery through the cortex and out through muscle attachments.

Remodeling, Growth and Development

Bone Resorption and Renewal

Whereas renewal in tissues such as muscle occurs largely at a molecular level, renewal of bone occurs at a tissue level and is similar to the remodeling of buildings in that local removal (resorption) of old bone must precede new bone deposition. Remodeling is most vigorous during the years of active growth, when deposition predominates over resorption. Thereafter remodeling gradually declines, in humans until about age 35, after which its rate remains unchanged or increases slightly. From the fourth decade on, resorption exceeds formation, resulting in an approximate 10 percent loss in bone mass per decade, equivalent to a daily loss of 15 to 30 mg of calcium.

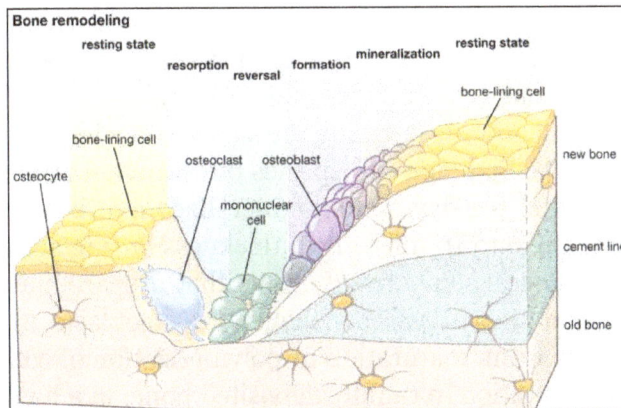

Bone Remodelling.

Except for the addition of the ossification mechanisms within cartilage, growth and development involve exactly the same type of remodeling as that in the adult skeleton. Both require continuous, probably irreversible differentiation of osteoclasts and osteoblasts, the former from circulating monocytes in the blood and the latter from the undifferentiated bone mesenchyme. The life span of osteoclasts is from a few hours to at most a few days, while that of osteoblasts is a few days to at most a few weeks.

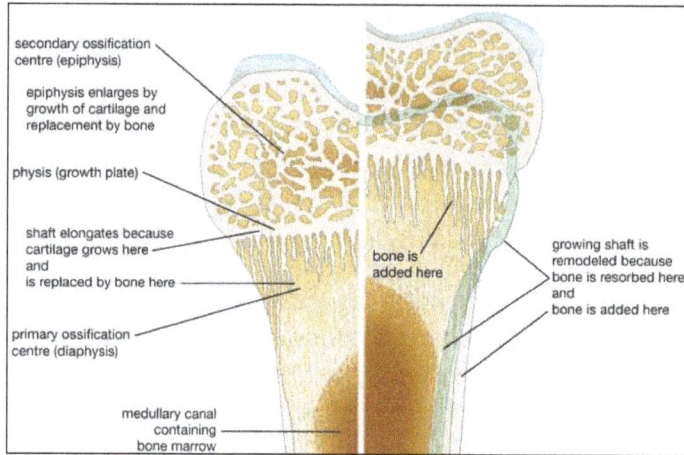

Bone remodeling.
Bone remodeling and growth.

Resorption is produced by clusters of osteoclasts that either erode free bone surfaces or form "cutting cones" that tunnel through compact bone and create the cylindrical cavities that may be subsequently filled by osteons. Osteoclastic cells secrete enzymes and hydrogen ions onto the bone surface, dissolving the mineral and digesting the matrix at virtually the same moment. The process is associated with locally augmented blood flow and with a greater surface acidity than elsewhere in bone, despite the fact that the process of dissolving apatite consumes hydrogen ions. Resorption is usually a much more rapid process than formation. Osteoclastic cutting cones have been observed to advance at rates up to 500 micrometres, or microns, per day (1 micron = 1×10^{-6} metre).

Bone is formed on previously resorbed surfaces by deposition of an unmineralized protein matrix material (osteoid) and its subsequent mineralization. Osteoblasts elaborate matrix as a continuous membrane covering the surface on which they are working at a linear rate that varies with both age and species but which in large adult mammals is on the order of one micron per day. The unmineralized matrix constitutes an osteoid seam or border, averaging 6 to 10 microns in thickness during active bone formation. The biochemical and physical sequence of events that prepare matrix for mineralization includes intracellular biosynthesis of collagen by osteoblasts, extrusion of collagen extracellularly in soluble form, maturation or polymerization of collagen into an array of fibrils (in random orientation in rapidly deposited bone, in a highly ordered regular pattern in slowly formed lamellar bone), binding of calcium to collagen fibrils, and formation of protein-glycoaminoglycan complexes.

Mineralization itself depends upon establishment of crystal nuclei within the matrix; this process requires 5 to 10 days and is under the control of the osteoblast, but its exact chemistry is obscure. A suitable nucleating configuration is somehow established, and, once nuclei reach a critical size, further mineralization proceeds spontaneously in the presence of usual body fluid calcium and phosphorus concentrations. Other collagenous tissues, such as dermis, tendon, and ligament, do not normally calcify, even though bathed by the same body fluids as bone. Although extracellular fluid is a highly supersaturated solution with respect to hydroxylapatite, calcium and phosphorus will not spontaneously precipitate in this crystalline form at normal physiological pH, so one and the same fluid is indefinitely stable in non-bone-forming regions yet richly supports mineralization in the presence of suitable crystal nuclei. Mineral movement into new bone is initially rapid and in compact bone is known to reach approximately 70 percent of full mineralization within a few hours after matrix nucleation. This mineral deposition involves replacement of the water that occupied half the original matrix volume. As water content decreases, further mineral diffusion is impeded; and the final mineralization occurs progressively more slowly over a period of many weeks. In normal adult humans, new bone formation takes up about 400 mg of calcium per day, an amount approximately equal to that in the circulating blood.

Osteocytes, once thought of as resting cells, are now recognized to be metabolically active and to possess, at least in latent form, the ability to resorb and re-form bone on their lacunar walls. Although osteocytes constitute only a small fraction of total bone volume, they are so arranged within bone, and the network of their protoplasmic extensions is so extensive, that there is essentially no volume of bony material situated more than a fraction of a micron from a cell or its processes. Of the more than 1,200 square metres (1,435 square yards) of anatomic surface within the skeleton of an adult man, about 99 percent is accounted for by the lacunar and canalicular surfaces. Resorption and deposition on this surface serve both to regulate plasma calcium concentration and to renew bony material. This renewal may be particularly important because all composite materials change in their physical properties with time. It is not known whether bone properties change sufficiently to have biological consequence, but, to the extent that such change does occur, renewal around osteocytes would provide for the physical maintenance of bone structural material.

Types of Bone Formation

Bone is formed in the embryo in two general ways. For most bones the general shape is first laid down as a cartilage model, which is then progressively replaced by bone (endochondral bone formation). A few bones (such as the clavicle and the calvarium) develop within a condensed region of fibrous tissue without a cartilaginous intermediate (membrane bone formation). In long bones a collar of spongy membrane bone is first laid down in the fibrous tissues surrounding the cartilaginous model of the shaft. At the same time, the cartilage deep to this collar begins to degenerate and calcify. The bone is then penetrated by blood vessels, which grow into the degenerating model and remove the calcified cartilage enclosed within the collar. Vascular invasion proceeds toward both ends of the model in parallel with continued extension of the bony collar. This leaves a structure consisting of two cartilaginous epiphyses at the ends of a hollow bony shaft.

Growth from this point on is accomplished in two ways. Radial growth occurs by deposition of new bone on the periosteal surface and roughly equivalent resorption at the endosteal surface. Longitudinal growth involves replacement of cartilage by bone from the shaft side of the growth plate, at a rate closely matched by the rate of production of new cartilage by the plate itself. The growth plate consists of highly ordered rows of cartilage cells; the row farthest removed from the bony shaft is a basal or germinal layer, responsible for cell replication and cartilage growth. The complex sequence of longitudinal growth consists of cartilage cell degeneration farthest from the germinal layer, calcification of cartilage in that area, deposition over it of a thin layer of true bone (primary spongiosa), and, finally, osteoclastic resorption to extend the medullary cavity in parallel with longitudinal growth and to reshape the contour of the shaft.

This process of cartilage growth, degeneration, calcification, and ultimate replacement by bone is responsible for most growth in length in vertebrates. It first begins in the embryo and continues until full skeletal maturity, when in most species the growth plates fuse and disappear.

The appearance of epiphyseal ossification centres and their ultimate fusion, both of which can be detected by ordinary X-rays, normally follow an orderly and predictable sequence that is of great value in the evaluation of disorders of growth and development. Because of the complicated interaction of several tissue elements in the process of endochondral ossification, the metaphyseal region of bones is the seat of, or prominently reflects, many nutritional or metabolic disturbances of growth. Examples of disorders involving this growth mechanism include rickets and achondroplastic dwarfism.

Physiology of Bone

Calcium and Phosphate Equilibrium

As important as the structural properties of bone is the role bone plays in the maintenance of the ionic composition of the blood and interstitial fluids of the body. All vertebrates possessing true bone exhibit body-fluid calcium ion concentrations of approximately 50 mg per litre (1.25 millimoles) and phosphorus concentrations in the range of 30–100 mg per litre (1–3 millimoles). These levels, particularly those of calcium, are extremely important for the maintenance of normal neuromuscular function, interneuronal transmission, cell membrane integrity and permeability, and blood coagulation. The rigid constancy with which calcium levels are maintained, both in the individual and throughout all higher vertebrate classes, attests to the biological importance of such regulation. Approximately 99 percent of total body calcium and 85 percent of total body phosphorus reside in the mineral deposits of bone; thus, bone is quantitatively in a position to mediate adjustments in concentration of these two ions in the circulating body fluids. Such adjustments are provided by three hormonal control loops (control systems with feedback) and by at least three locally acting mechanisms. The hormonal loops involve parathyroid hormone (PTH), calcitonin (CT), and vitamin D and are concerned exclusively with regulation of calcium ion and phosphorus ion concentrations.

PTH and vitamin D act to elevate ionized calcium levels in body fluids, and CT (from the ultimobranchial body or C cells of the thyroid gland) acts to depress them. The secretion of each hormone is controlled by the level of calcium ion in the circulating blood. At normal calcium concentrations, there are low levels of secretion of all three hormones. When the blood levels of ionized calcium decline, there is an almost immediate increase in PTH synthesis and secretion. PTH has three principal actions in maintaining blood calcium concentrations. It directly stimulates the kidneys to enhance the tubular reabsorption of calcium from the ultrafiltrate that would otherwise be excreted into the urine. It also stimulates the kidney to activate the major circulating form of vitamin D to calcitrial. Calcitrial enters the circulation and travels to the small intestine where it acts to increase the absorption efficiency of dietary calcium into the bloodstream.

PTH and calcitrial can also stimulate osteoblasts to produce osteoclast differentiation factor (ODF). Osteoblasts that have ODF on their surfaces can interact with the precursor cells of osteoclasts (monocytes) to induce them to become mature osteoclasts. The osteoclasts in turn release hydrochloric acid and enzymes into the mineralized bone and release calcium and phosphorus into the circulation. Thus, when there is inadequate dietary calcium to satisfy the body's calcium needs, both PTH and calcitrial work in concert on osteoblasts to recruit precursors of osteoclasts to become mature osteoclasts. When the body's calcium needs are satisfied by adequate dietary intake of calcium, both PTH and calcitrial act on osteoblasts to increase their activity, resulting in increased bone formation and mineralization. Calcitonin is the only hormone that interacts directly on osteoclasts, which have a receptor for it. It decreases mature osteoclastic activity, thereby inhibiting their function.

PTH and calcitrial also are important in maintaining serum phosphorus levels. PTH interferes with renal tubular phosphorus reabsorption, causing an enhanced renal excretion of phosphorus. This mechanism, which serves to lower levels of phosphorus in the bloodstream, is significant because high phosphate levels inhibit and low levels enhance osteoclastic reabsorption. Calcium ion itself has similar effects on the osteoclastic process: high levels inhibit and low levels enhance the effect of systemically acting agents such as PTH. On the other hand, PTH stimulates the production of calcitrial, which in turn stimulates the small intestine to increase its efficacy of absorption of dietary phosphorus.

A deficiency in vitamin D results in poor mineralization of the skeleton, causing rickets in children and osteomalacia in adults. Mineralization defects are due to the decrease in the efficiency of intestinal calcium absorption, which results in a decrease in ionized calcium concentrations in blood. This results in an increase in PTH in the circulation, which increases serum calcium and decreases serum phosphorus because of the enhanced excretion of phosphorus into the urine.

The exact function of calcitonin is not fully understood. However, it can offset elevations in high calcium ion levels by decreasing osteoclast activity, resulting in inhibition of bone absorption.

Physiological and Mechanical Controls

In the language of control mechanics, remodeling depends upon two control loops with negative feedback: a homeostatic loop involving the effects of PTH and CT on resorption and a mechanical loop that brings about changes in skeletal mass and arrangement to meet changing structural needs. The PTH-CT loop is basically a systemic process, and the mechanical loop is local; however, the two loops interact significantly at the level of the cells that act as intermediaries in both processes. A large number of other factors, including minerals in the diet, hormonal balance, disease, and aging, have important effects on the skeleton that interact with the control system.

The controls exerted by mechanical forces, recognized for over a century, have been formulated as Wolff's law: "Every change in the function of a bone is followed by certain definite changes in its internal architecture and its external conformation." Of the many theories proposed to explain how mechanical forces communicate with the cells responsible for bone formation and resorption, the most appealing has been postulation of induced local electrical fields that mediate this information exchange. Many crystalline or semicrystalline materials, including both bone collagen and its associated mineral, exhibit piezoelectric properties. Deformation of macroscopic units of bone by mechanical force produces a charge in the millivolt range and current flow on the order of 10^{-15} ampere; both voltage and current flow are proportional to the applied force. Regions under tension act as anode and compressed regions as cathode. Currents of this magnitude are capable of aligning collagen fibrils as they aggregate from the solution phase and are known also to alter the cell-based development of regeneration buds in amphibia. The negative feedback characteristic of this mechanism lies in the fact that bone accumulates about the cathodal region of this system, hence reducing the electrical effects produced by an applied force.

The mechanisms by which the bone mesenchyme responds to mechanical stimuli (whether or not mediated by electrical signals) are uncertain. In general, heavy usage leads to heavy bone, and disuse, as in immobilization associated with injury or severe disease, results in decreased bone mass and increased excretion of calcium, phosphorus, and nitrogen. The cellular response, however, is discouragingly complex. In broad outline it appears that the local expression of decreased stress is an increase in bone resorption coupled variably with a smaller and secondary increase in bone formation, whereas increased stress appears to be accompanied by a decrease in bone resorption coupled also with a smaller and probably secondary increase in bone formation. The decrease in resorption represents a decreased sensitivity to systemic stimuli, such as PTH, and reflects an interaction between hormonal and physical forces at the cellular level. PTH is the major determinant of all remodeling, structural as well as homeostatic; mechanical forces are the major determinant of where that remodeling occurs.

One of the most arresting features of skeletal remodeling is the tendency for rates of bone resorption and bone formation to change in the same direction. Three mechanisms for this coupling can be identified. The first is homeostatic and rises from the mineral demand created by formation of crystal nuclei in the bone matrix. Unless the calcium demands of increased bone formation can be met by some other source (such as an increase in calcium in the diet), they will inevitably lead to increased PTH secretion and bone resorption. Since the level of PTH is a principal determinant of bone resorption, it follows that high levels of formation tend to produce high levels of resorption (and vice versa). A second mechanism is the mechanical force–piezoelectric system. Local bone resorption, by reducing structural volume, concentrates applied forces in the remaining bone; this leads to increased strain and presumably increases the stimulus for local bone repair. A third mechanism is inferred from the observation in adult animals that the induction of specialized bony cells from the mesenchyme proceeds in a predetermined sequence—first osteoclasts and then osteoblasts—so that, even on free surfaces, resorption usually precedes formation. The ultimate basis of this cellular coupling is not known.

Hormonal Influences

The most striking effects of estrogens are seen in birds. During the part of the life cycle prior to egg formation, a marked increase in osteoblastic activity occurs along the inside surfaces of the long bones, and the medullary cavities become filled with spongy bone. As the egg is formed, this spongy bone is rapidly resorbed; plasma calcium rises dramatically; and calcium is deposited in the shell. In mammals studied prior to skeletal maturity, administration of estrogens produces an accelerated appearance of ossification centres, a slowing in growth of cartilage and bone, and fusion of the epiphyses; the result is an adult skeleton smaller than normal. In older mammals, estrogens in certain dosages and schedules of administration may inhibit trabecular bone resorption, and, in some species, prolonged administration of estrogen may lead to increased bone porosity. In postmenopausal women, administration of estrogen suppresses bone resorption and produces a transient decrease in serum calcium and phosphorus and in renal reabsorption of phosphorus, as well as positive calcium balance—effects that help to stabilize the total skeletal bone mass.

The effects described are for estrogens as a general class of steroid hormones, and no attempt has been made to differentiate between the actions of natural estrogenic hormones and the many synthetic varieties now in wide use to suppress ovulation.

Very little is known of the effects of progesterone on bone beyond studies in young guinea pigs suggesting slight inhibition of the activity of such hormones as estrogens, which speed skeletal development.

In mammals, including humans, just prior to sexual maturity, the growth spurt occurring in males is attributable principally to the growth-promoting action of the male sex hormone testosterone. When administered, testosterone and related steroids stimulate linear growth for a limited period; ultimately, however, particularly if they are given in large doses, they suppress bone growth as the result of hastened skeletal development and premature epiphyseal closure. Studies have indicated that testosterone derivatives administered to adult mammals suppress the turnover and resorption of bone and increase the retention of nitrogen, phosphorus, and calcium.

The influence of the adrenal corticosteroid hormones on bone is varied, but the principal result is slowing of growth in the young and decrease in bone mass in the adult. In Cushing syndrome, in which there is abnormally high secretion of corticosteroids, bone loss to the point of fractures often occurs. Cortisol in high concentration suppresses protein and mucopolysaccharide synthesis, with inhibition of bone matrix formation and of incorporation of nucleosides into bone cells. Cortisol also inhibits intestinal calcium absorption, which in turn causes increases in PTH production and the rate of bone resorption.

Lack of the internal secretion of the thyroid gland results in retardation of skeletal growth and development. Action of this hormone to facilitate growth and skeletal maturation is probably indirect, through its general effects on cell metabolism. Thyroid hormone in excess leads in the young to premature appearance of ossification centres and closure of the epiphyses and in adults to increased bone-cell metabolism. Commonly, in the hyperthyroid adult, bone resorption predominates over increased bone formation with resultant loss of bone mass.

The anterior lobe of the pituitary gland secretes a hormone essential for growth and development of the skeleton. This effect of the hormone is indirect and mediated by "sulfation factor," a substance produced in the liver in response to stimulation by the growth hormone. The extent to which growth hormone is involved in skeletal remodeling in the adult is not known, but excessive elaboration of the hormone after maturity leads to distorted enlargement of all bones in the condition known as acromegaly. Excessive elaboration of growth hormone prior to epiphyseal closure leads to gigantism. Studies of the administration of growth hormone to humans have indicated marked species specificity; growth in hypopituitary dwarfs is stimulated only by human or primate growth hormone. The principal metabolic effects of the hormone in humans are retention of nitrogen and increased turnover of calcium, resulting in increases both in intestinal calcium absorption and in urinary calcium excretion.

Insulin participates in the regulation of bone growth; it may enhance or even be necessary for the effect of growth hormone on bone. Insulin has been found to stimulate growth and epiphyseal widening in rats whose pituitaries have been removed and to promote chondroitin sulfate synthesis in cartilage and bone and the transport of amino acids and nucleosides into bone.

Nutritional Influences

The most significant nutritional influence on bone is the availability of calcium. The close relationship between bone and calcium is indicated by the principal processes of calcium metabolism. Bone contains 99 percent of the calcium in the body and can behave as an adequate buffer for maintenance of a constant level of freely moving calcium in soft tissues, extracellular fluid, and blood. The free-calcium concentration in this pool must be kept within fairly narrow limits (50–65 mg per litre of extracellular fluid) to maintain the constant internal environment necessary for neuromuscular irritability, blood clotting, muscle contractility, and cardiac function. Calcium leaves the pool by way of bone formation, by such routes as the urine, feces, and sweat, and periodically by way of lactation and transplacental movement. Calcium enters the pool by the mechanism of bone resorption and by absorption from dietary calcium in the upper intestinal tract.

The significance with respect to bone of adequate availability of calcium to animals or humans is that the mechanical strength of bone is proportional to its mineral content. All of the other components of bone, organic and inorganic, are of course also essential for bone integrity, but the importance of availability of structural materials is most easily illustrated by consideration of calcium balance (dietary intake versus excretory output). If intake of calcium is limited, maintenance of normal levels of extracellular and soft tissue calcium in the face of mandatory daily losses from this pool by various excretory routes requires that calcium be mined from its storage depot, bone. Abundant mineral intake then tends to preserve bone mass, and an increase of positivity of calcium balance has been shown to suppress resorption of bone.

The Food and Nutrition Board of the U.S. National Academy of Sciences has recommended 1,000 to 2,000 mg of calcium daily for adults and 800 to 1,300 mg for children. The usual daily intake of calcium in the diet, however, is between 400 and 600 mg, about 150 to 250 mg from green vegetables and the remainder usually from milk and milk products. Daily urinary excretion of calcium is normally from 50 to 150 mg in females and 50 to 300 mg in males. Fecal excretion of calcium is much larger than urinary excretion; most of the calcium in the feces is unabsorbed dietary calcium. Heavy sweating can result in a loss of more than 200 mg per day. Calcium absorption varies depending on previous and current levels of calcium intake and type of diet. Approximately 30 percent of dietary calcium is absorbed when there is adequate vitamin D intake.

The other principal mineral constituent of bone is phosphorus, which is abundantly available in milk, meat, and other protein-rich foods. The recommended daily intake of phosphorus is 700 mg daily for adults, 1,250 mg daily for adolescents, and 500 mg daily for children up to age eight. A prolonged dietary deficiency in phosphorus or marked loss of phosphorus in the urine can result in mineral-poor bone, known as rickets in children and osteomalacia in adults. The skeleton also serves as a storage reservoir for magnesium. Magnesium deficiency can result in neuromuscular dysfunction similar to a calcium deficiency. Magnesium is critically important for the regulation of parathyroid hormone.

Fluoride, an element of proven value and safety in prevention of dental cavities when provided in drinking water at concentrations of one part per million, is absorbed into bone lattice structure as well as into enamel and produces a larger crystal more resistant to resorption. Amounts 10 or more times that normally taken in fluoridated drinking water have been noted to cause abnormalities of bone collagen synthesis. Extremely large dosages in humans produce the denser but irregularly structured and brittle bone of fluorosis.

The function of vitamin A remains to be clarified, but it is apparently necessary for proliferation of cartilage and bone growth. Without vitamin A, bone remodeling is also impaired and bones develop in abnormal shapes. Excessive amounts of the vitamin result in thinning of cortical bone and fracture.

Ascorbic acid, or vitamin C, is essential for intracellular formation of collagen and for hydroxylation of proline. In scurvy, a disease caused by vitamin C deficiency, the collagen matrix of bone is either partially or completely unable to calcify.

Vitamin D has several complex physiologic actions that affect calcium, phosphorus, and bone metabolism. A form of vitamin D called calcitrial increases the efficiency of intestinal calcium absorption and also interacts directly with osteoblasts to increase osteoblast function. At times when dietary calcium is inadequate, calcitrial will stimulate osteoblasts to increase osteoclast differentiation factor (ODF) on their surface, which in turn mobilizes osteoclast mesenchymal cells to become mature osteoclasts. Thus, the major function of vitamin D is to maintain serum levels of calcium by increasing absorption of dietary calcium in the intestine. At times of increased need, such as during pregnancy, lactation, and adolescent growth, circulating levels of calcitrial are increased, resulting in an increase of up to 80 percent in the efficiency of intestinal calcium absorption. In vitamin D deficiency, parathyroid hormone levels are elevated, causing an increased loss of phosphorus into the urine.

Other nutritional factors include protein, which, as an essential component of the matrix of bone, must be provided by a combination of dietary intake and conversion from other tissues. Changes in acid-base balance also have an influence on the skeleton—acidosis in various clinical disorders and ingestion of acid salts being accompanied by mineral loss.

MUSCLE

Muscle is a soft tissue found in most animals. Muscle cells contain protein filaments of actin and myosin that slide past one another, producing a contraction that changes both the length and the shape of the cell. Muscles function to produce force and motion. They are primarily responsible for maintaining and changing posture, locomotion, as well as movement of internal organs, such as the contraction of the heart and the movement of food through the digestive system via peristalsis.

Muscle tissues are derived from the mesodermal layer of embryonic germ cells in a process known as myogenesis. There are three types of muscle, skeletal or striated, cardiac, and smooth. Muscle action can be classified as being either voluntary or involuntary. Cardiac and smooth muscles contract without conscious thought and are termed involuntary, whereas the skeletal muscles contract upon command. Skeletal muscles in turn can be divided into fast and slow twitch fibers.

Muscles are predominantly powered by the oxidation of fats and carbohydrates, but anaerobic chemical reactions are also used, particularly by fast twitch fibers. These chemical reactions produce adenosine triphosphate (ATP) molecules that are used to power the movement of the myosin heads.

Structure

The anatomy of muscles includes gross anatomy, which comprises all the muscles of an organism, and microanatomy, which comprises the structures of a single muscle.

Types

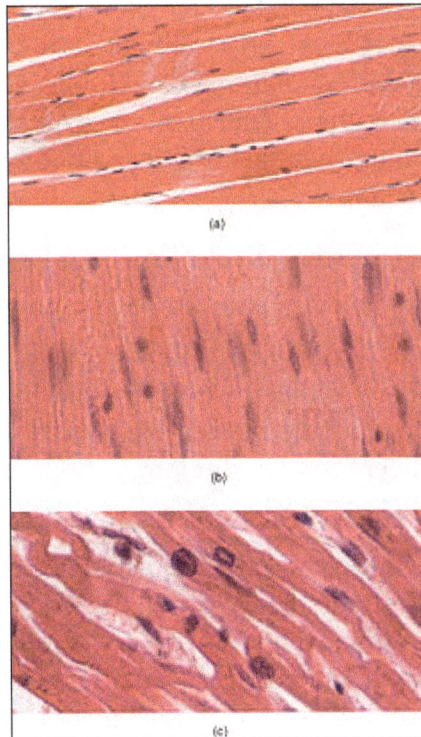

(a)

(b)

(c)

The body contains three types of muscle tissue: (a) skeletal muscle, (b) smooth muscle, and (c) cardiac muscle. (Same magnification)

Muscle tissue is a soft tissue, and is one of the four fundamental types of tissue present in animals. There are three types of muscle tissue recognized in vertebrates:

- Skeletal muscle or "voluntary muscle" is anchored by tendons (or by aponeuroses at a few places) to bone and is used to effect skeletal movement such as locomotion and in maintaining posture. Though this postural control is generally maintained as an unconscious reflex, the muscles responsible react to conscious control like non-postural muscles. An average adult male is made up of 42% of skeletal muscle and an average adult female is made up of 36% (as a percentage of body mass).

- Smooth muscle or "involuntary muscle" is found within the walls of organs and structures such as the esophagus, stomach, intestines, bronchi, uterus, urethra, bladder, blood vessels, and the arrector pili in the skin (in which it controls erection of body hair). Unlike skeletal muscle, smooth muscle is not under conscious control.

- Cardiac muscle (myocardium), is also an "involuntary muscle" but is more akin in structure to skeletal muscle, and is found only in the heart.

Cardiac and skeletal muscles are "striated" in that they contain sarcomeres that are packed into highly regular arrangements of bundles; the myofibrils of smooth muscle cells are not arranged in sarcomeres and so are not striated. While the sarcomeres in skeletal muscles are arranged in regular, parallel bundles, cardiac muscle sarcomeres connect at branching, irregular angles (called intercalated discs). Striated muscle contracts and relaxes in short, intense bursts, whereas smooth muscle sustains longer or even near-permanent contractions.

Skeletal (voluntary) muscle is further divided into two broad types: *slow twitch* and *fast twitch*:

- Type I, slow twitch, or "red" muscle, is dense with capillaries and is rich in mitochondria and myoglobin, giving the muscle tissue its characteristic red color. It can carry more oxygen and sustain aerobic activity using fats or carbohydrates as fuel. Slow twitch fibers contract for long periods of time but with little force.

- Type II, fast twitch muscle, has three major subtypes (IIa, IIx, and IIb) that vary in both contractile speed and force generated. Fast twitch fibers contract quickly and powerfully but fatigue very rapidly, sustaining only short, anaerobic bursts of activity before muscle contraction becomes painful. They contribute most to muscle strength and have greater potential for increase in mass. Type IIb is anaerobic, glycolytic, "white" muscle that is least dense in mitochondria and myoglobin. In small animals (e.g., rodents) this is the major fast muscle type, explaining the pale color of their flesh.

The density of mammalian skeletal muscle tissue is about 1.06 kg/liter. This can be contrasted with the density of adipose tissue (fat), which is 0.9196 kg/liter. This makes muscle tissue approximately 15% denser than fat tissue.

Microanatomy

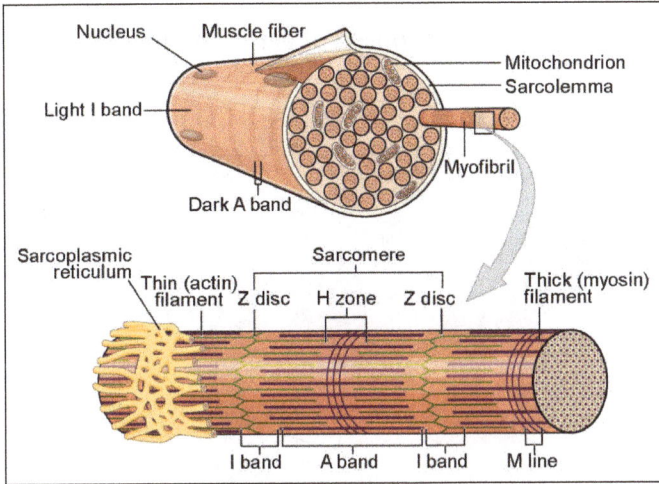

A skeletal muscle fiber is surrounded by a plasma membrane called the sarcolemma, which contains sarcoplasm, the cytoplasm of muscle cells. A muscle fiber is composed of many fibrils, which give the cell its striated appearance.

Skeletal muscles are sheathed by a tough layer of connective tissue called the epimysium. The epimysium anchors muscle tissue to tendons at each end, where the epimysium becomes thicker and collagenous. It also protects muscles from friction against other muscles and bones. Within the epimysium are multiple bundles called fascicles, each of which contains 10 to 100 or more muscle fibers collectively sheathed by a perimysium. Besides surrounding each fascicle, the perimysium is a pathway for nerves and the flow of blood within the muscle. The threadlike muscle fibers are the individual muscle cells (myocytes), and each cell is encased within its own endomysium of collagen fibers. Thus, the overall muscle consists of fibers (cells) that are bundled into fascicles, which are themselves grouped together to form muscles. At each level of bundling, a collagenous membrane surrounds the bundle, and these membranes support muscle function both by resisting passive stretching of the tissue and by distributing forces applied to the muscle. Scattered throughout the muscles are muscle spindles that provide sensory feedback information to the central nervous system. (This grouping structure is analogous to the organization of nerves which uses epineurium, perineurium, and endoneurium).

This same bundles-within-bundles structure is replicated within the muscle cells. Within the cells of the muscle are myofibrils, which themselves are bundles of protein filaments. The term "myofibril" should not be confused with "myofiber", which is a simply another name for a muscle cell. Myofibrils are complex strands of several kinds of protein filaments organized together into repeating units called sarcomeres. The striated appearance of both skeletal and cardiac muscle results from the regular pattern of sarcomeres within their cells. Although both of these types of muscle contain sarcomeres, the fibers in cardiac muscle are typically branched to form a network. Cardiac muscle fibers are interconnected by intercalated discs, giving that tissue the appearance of a syncytium.

The filaments in a sarcomere are composed of actin and myosin.

Gross Anatomy

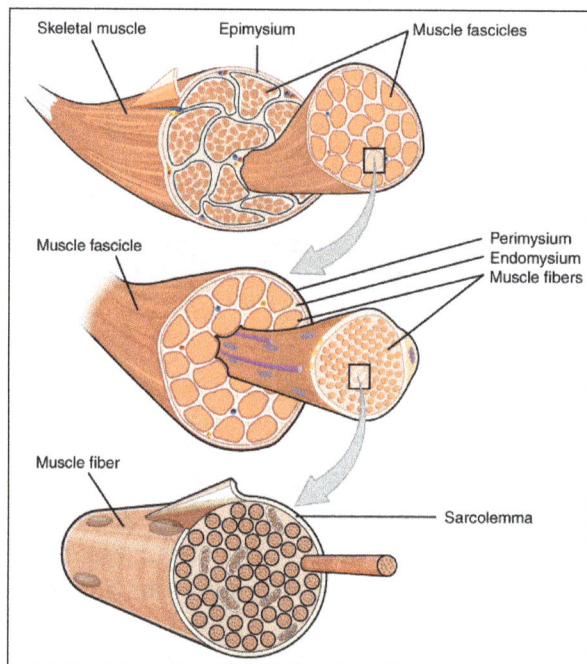

Bundles of muscle fibers, called fascicles, are covered by the perimysium.
Muscle fibers are covered by the endomysium.

The gross anatomy of a muscle is the most important indicator of its role in the body. There is an important distinction seen between pennate muscles and other muscles. In most muscles, all the fibers are oriented in the same direction, running in a line from the origin to the insertion. However, In pennate muscles, the individual fibers are oriented at an angle relative to the line of action, attaching to the origin and insertion tendons at each end. Because the contracting fibers are pulling at an angle to the overall action of the muscle, the change in length is smaller, but this same orientation allows for more fibers (thus more force) in a muscle of a given size. Pennate muscles are usually found where their length change is less important than maximum force, such as the rectus femoris.

Skeletal muscle is arranged in discrete muscles, an example of which is the *biceps brachii* (biceps). The tough, fibrous epimysium of skeletal muscle is both connected to and continuous with the tendons. In turn, the tendons connect to the periosteum layer surrounding the bones, permitting the transfer of force from the muscles to the skeleton. Together, these fibrous layers, along with tendons and ligaments, constitute the deep fascia of the body.

Muscular System

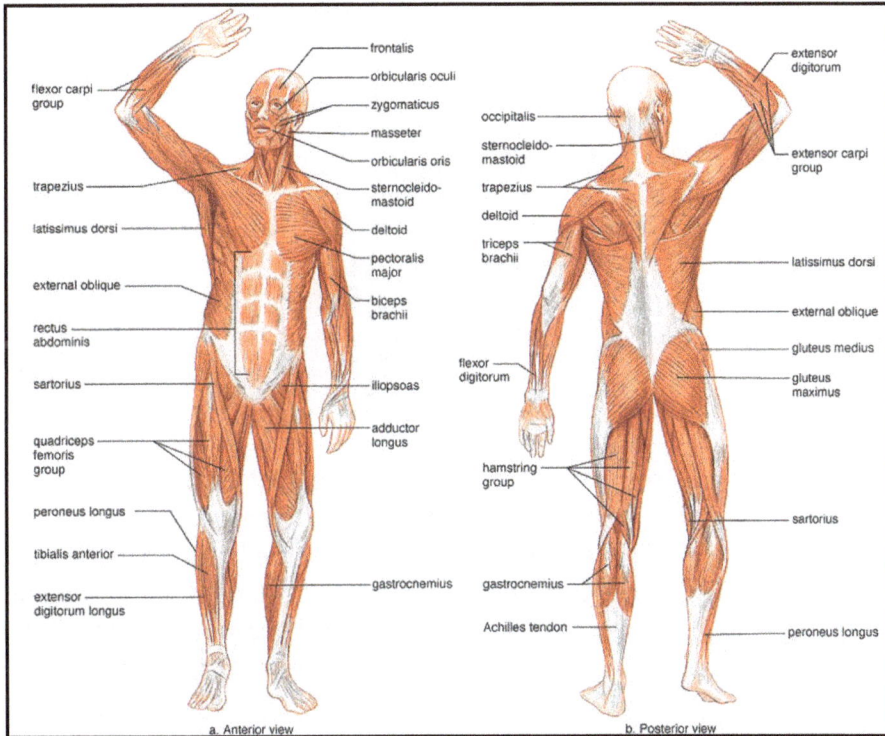

On the anterior and posterior views of the muscular system above, superficial muscles (those at the surface) are shown on the right side of the body while deep muscles (those underneath the superficial muscles) are shown on the left half of the body. For the legs, superficial muscles are shown in the anterior view while the posterior view shows both superficial and deep muscles.

The muscular system consists of all the muscles present in a single body. There are approximately 650 skeletal muscles in the human body, but an exact number is difficult to define. The difficulty lies partly in the fact that different sources group the muscles differently and partly in that some muscles, such as palmaris longus, are not always present.

A muscular *slip* is a narrow length of muscle that acts to augment a larger muscle or muscles.

The muscular system is one component of the musculoskeletal system, which includes not only the muscles but also the bones, joints, tendons, and other structures that permit movement.

Development

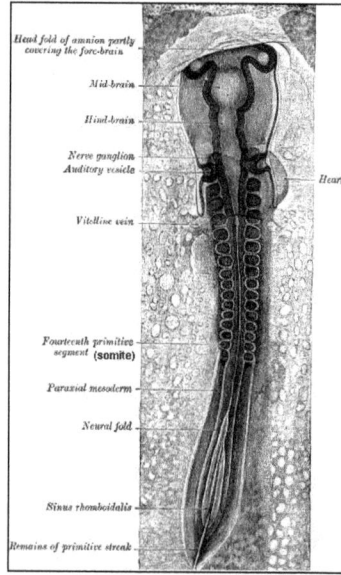

All muscles are derived from paraxial mesoderm. The paraxial mesoderm is divided along the embryo's length into somites, corresponding to the segmentation of the body (most obviously seen in the vertebral column. Each somite has 3 divisions, sclerotome (which forms vertebrae), dermatome (which forms skin), and myotome (which forms muscle). The myotome is divided into two sections, the epimere and hypomere, which form epaxial and hypaxial muscles, respectively. The only epaxial muscles in humans are the erector spinae and small intervertebral muscles, and are innervated by the dorsal rami of the spinal nerves. All other muscles, including those of the limbs are hypaxial, and inervated by the ventral rami of the spinal nerves.

During development, myoblasts (muscle progenitor cells) either remain in the somite to form muscles associated with the vertebral column or migrate out into the body to form all other muscles. Myoblast migration is preceded by the formation of connective tissue frameworks, usually formed from the somatic lateral plate mesoderm. Myoblasts follow chemical signals to the appropriate locations, where they fuse into elongate skeletal muscle cells.

Physiology

Contraction

The three types of muscle (skeletal, cardiac and smooth) have significant differences. However, all three use the movement of actin against myosin to create contraction.

In skeletal muscle, contraction is stimulated by electrical impulses transmitted by the nerves, the motoneurons (motor nerves) in particular. Cardiac and smooth muscle contractions are stimulated by internal pacemaker cells which regularly contract, and propagate contractions to other muscle cells they are in contact with. All skeletal muscle and many smooth muscle contractions are facilitated by the neurotransmitter acetylcholine.

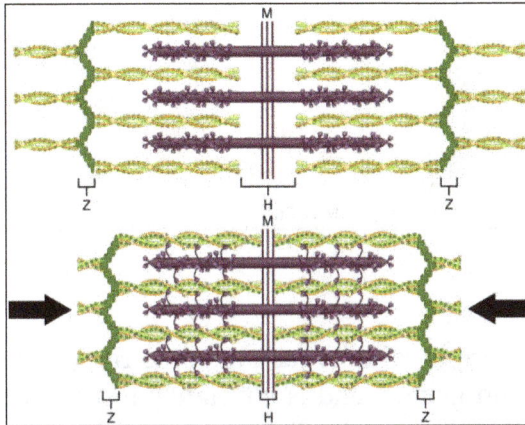

When a sarcomere contracts, the Z lines move closer together, and the I band becomes smaller. The A band stays the same width. At full contraction, the thin and thick filaments overlap.

The action a muscle generates is determined by the origin and insertion locations. The cross-sectional area of a muscle (rather than volume or length) determines the amount of force it can generate by defining the number of "sarcomeres" which can operate in parallel. Each skeletal muscle contains long units called myofibrils, and each myofibril is a chain of sarcomeres. Since contraction occurs at the same time for all connected sarcomeres in a muscles cell, these chains of sarcomeres shorten together, thus shortening the muscle fiber, resulting in overall length change. The amount of force applied to the external environment is determined by lever mechanics, specifically the ratio of in-lever to out-lever. For example, moving the insertion point of the biceps more distally on the radius (farther from the joint of rotation) would increase the force generated during flexion (and, as a result, the maximum weight lifted in this movement), but decrease the maximum speed of flexion. Moving the insertion point proximally (closer to the joint of rotation) would result in decreased force but increased velocity. This can be most easily seen by comparing the limb of a mole to a horse—in the former, the insertion point is positioned to maximize force (for digging), while in the latter, the insertion point is positioned to maximize speed (for running).

Nervous Control

Simplified schema of basic nervous system function. Signals are picked up by sensory receptors and sent to the spinal cord and brain via the afferent leg of the peripheral nervous system, whereupon processing occurs that results in signals sent back to the spinal cord and then out to motor neurons via the efferent leg.

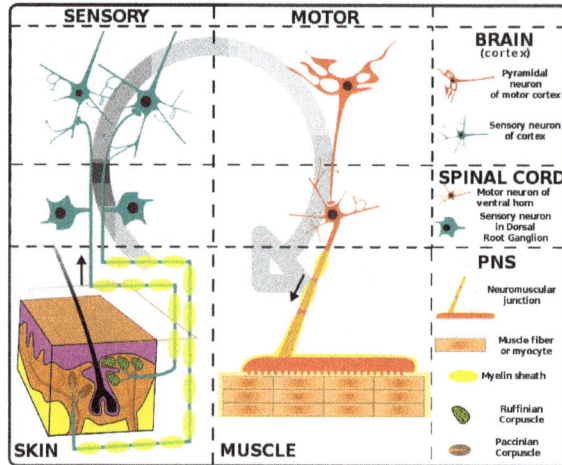

Muscle Movement

The efferent leg of the peripheral nervous system is responsible for conveying commands to the muscles and glands, and is ultimately responsible for voluntary movement. Nerves move muscles in response to voluntary and autonomic (involuntary) signals from the brain. Deep muscles, superficial muscles, muscles of the face and internal muscles all correspond with dedicated regions in the primary motor cortex of the brain, directly anterior to the central sulcus that divides the frontal and parietal lobes.

In addition, muscles react to reflexive nerve stimuli that do not always send signals all the way to the brain. In this case, the signal from the afferent fiber does not reach the brain, but produces the reflexive movement by direct connections with the efferent nerves in the spine. However, the majority of muscle activity is volitional, and the result of complex interactions between various areas of the brain.

Nerves that control skeletal muscles in mammals correspond with neuron groups along the primary motor cortex of the brain's cerebral cortex. Commands are routed though the basal ganglia and are modified by input from the cerebellum before being relayed through the pyramidal tract to the spinal cord and from there to the motor end plate at the muscles. Along the way, feedback, such as that of the extrapyramidal system contribute signals to influence muscle tone and response.

Deeper muscles such as those involved in posture often are controlled from nuclei in the brain stem and basal ganglia.

Proprioception

In skeletal muscles, muscle spindles convey information about the degree of muscle length and stretch to the central nervous system to assist in maintaining posture and joint position. The sense of where our bodies are in space is called proprioception, the perception of body awareness, the "unconscious" awareness of where the various regions of the body are located at any one time. Several areas in the brain coordinate movement and position with the feedback information gained from proprioception. The cerebellum and red nucleus in particular continuously sample position against movement and make minor corrections to assure smooth motion.

Energy Consumption

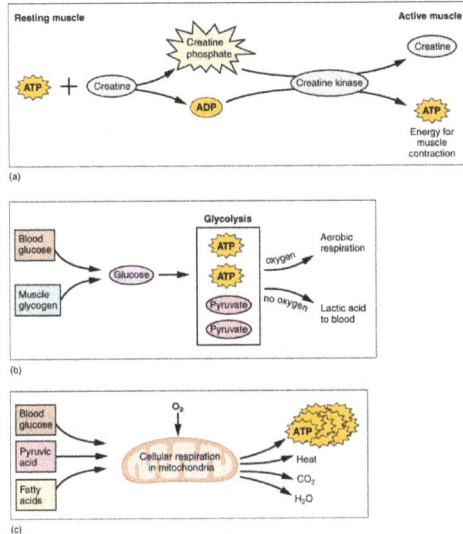

(a) Some ATP is stored in a resting muscle. As contraction starts, it is used up in seconds. More ATP is generated from creatine phosphate for about 15 seconds. (b) Each glucose molecule produces two ATP and two molecules of pyruvic acid, which can be used in aerobic respiration or converted to lactic acid. If oxygen is not available, pyruvic acid is converted to lactic acid, which may contribute to muscle fatigue. This occurs during strenuous exercise when high amounts of energy are needed but oxygen cannot be sufficiently delivered to muscle. (c) Aerobic respiration is the breakdown of glucose in the presence of oxygen (O_2) to produce carbon dioxide, water, and ATP. Approximately 95 percent of the ATP required for resting or moderately active muscles is provided by aerobic respiration, which takes place in mitochondria.

Muscular activity accounts for much of the body's energy consumption. All muscle cells produce adenosine triphosphate (ATP) molecules which are used to power the movement of the myosin heads. Muscles have a short-term store of energy in the form of creatine phosphate which is generated from ATP and can regenerate ATP when needed with creatine kinase. Muscles also keep a storage form of glucose in the form of glycogen. Glycogen can be rapidly converted to glucose when energy is required for sustained, powerful contractions. Within the voluntary skeletal muscles, the glucose molecule can be metabolized anaerobically in a process called glycolysis which produces two ATP and two lactic acid molecules in the process (note that in aerobic conditions, lactate is not formed; instead pyruvate is formed and transmitted through the citric acid cycle). Muscle cells also contain globules of fat, which are used for energy during aerobic exercise. The aerobic energy systems take longer to produce the ATP and reach peak efficiency, and requires many more biochemical steps, but produces significantly more ATP than anaerobic glycolysis. Cardiac muscle on the other hand, can readily consume any of the three macronutrients (protein, glucose and fat) aerobically without a 'warm up' period and always extracts the maximum ATP yield from any molecule involved. The heart, liver and red blood cells will also consume lactic acid produced and excreted by skeletal muscles during exercise.

At rest, skeletal muscle consumes 54.4 kJ/kg (13.0 kcal/kg) per day. This is larger than adipose tissue (fat) at 18.8 kJ/kg (4.5 kcal/kg), and bone at 9.6 kJ/kg (2.3 kcal/kg).

Efficiency

The efficiency of human muscle has been measured (in the context of rowing and cycling) at 18% to 26%. The efficiency is defined as the ratio of mechanical work output to the total metabolic cost, as can be calculated from oxygen consumption. This low efficiency is the result of about 40% efficiency of generating ATP from food energy, losses in converting energy from ATP into mechanical work inside the muscle, and mechanical losses inside the body. The latter two losses are dependent on the type of exercise and the type of muscle fibers being used (fast-twitch or slow-twitch). For an overall efficiency of 20 percent, one watt of mechanical power is equivalent to 4.3 kcal per hour. For example, one manufacturer of rowing equipment calibrates its rowing ergometer to count burned calories as equal to four times the actual mechanical work, plus 300 kcal per hour, this amounts to about 20 percent efficiency at 250 watts of mechanical output. The mechanical energy output of a cyclic contraction can depend upon many factors, including activation timing, muscle strain trajectory, and rates of force rise & decay. These can be synthesized experimentally using work loop analysis.

Strength

Muscle is a result of three factors that overlap: *physiological strength* (muscle size, cross sectional area, available crossbridging, responses to training), *neurological strength* (how strong or weak is the signal that tells the muscle to contract), and *mechanical strength* (muscle's force angle on the lever, moment arm length, joint capabilities).

Physiological Strength

Grading of muscle strength	
Grade 0	No contraction.

Grade 1	Trace of contraction, but no movement at the joint.
Grade 2	Movement at the joint with gravity eliminated.
Grade 3	Movement against gravity, but not against added resistance.
Grade 4	Movement against external resistance, but less than normal.
Grade 5	Normal strength.

Vertebrate muscle typically produces approximately 25–33 N (5.6–7.4 lb$_f$) of force per square centimeter of muscle cross-sectional area when isometric and at optimal length. Some invertebrate muscles, such as in crab claws, have much longer sarcomeres than vertebrates, resulting in many more sites for actin and myosin to bind and thus much greater force per square centimeter at the cost of much slower speed. The force generated by a contraction can be measured non-invasively using either mechanomyography or phonomyography, be measured in vivo using tendon strain (if a prominent tendon is present), or be measured directly using more invasive methods.

The strength of any given muscle, in terms of force exerted on the skeleton, depends upon length, shortening speed, cross sectional area, pennation, sarcomere length, myosin isoforms, and neural activation of motor units. Significant reductions in muscle strength can indicate underlying pathology, with the chart at right used as a guide.

The Strongest Human Muscle

Since three factors affect muscular strength simultaneously and muscles never work individually, it is misleading to compare strength in individual muscles, and state that one is the strongest. But below are several muscles whose strength is noteworthy for different reasons.

- In ordinary parlance, muscular "strength" usually refers to the ability to exert a force on an external object—for example, lifting a weight. By this definition, the masseter or jaw muscle is the strongest. The 1992 Guinness Book of Records records the achievement of a bite strength of 4,337 N (975 lb$_f$) for 2 seconds. What distinguishes the masseter is not anything special about the muscle itself, but its advantage in working against a much shorter lever arm than other muscles.

- If "strength" refers to the force exerted by the muscle itself, e.g., on the place where it inserts into a bone, then the strongest muscles are those with the largest cross-sectional area. This is because the tension exerted by an individual skeletal muscle fiber does not vary much. Each fiber can exert a force on the order of 0.3 micronewton. By this definition, the strongest muscle of the body is usually said to be the quadriceps femoris or the gluteus maximus.

- Because muscle strength is determined by cross-sectional area, a shorter muscle will be stronger "pound for pound" (i.e., by weight) than a longer muscle of the same cross-sectional area. The myometrial layer of the uterus may be the strongest muscle by weight in the female human body. At the time when an infant is delivered, the entire human uterus weighs about 1.1 kg (40 oz). During childbirth, the uterus exerts 100 to 400 N (25 to 100 lbf) of downward force with each contraction.

- The external muscles of the eye are conspicuously large and strong in relation to the small size and weight of the eyeball. It is frequently said that they are "the strongest muscles for the job they have to do" and are sometimes claimed to be "100 times stronger than they need to be." However, eye movements (particularly saccades used on facial scanning and reading) do require high speed movements, and eye muscles are exercised nightly during rapid eye movement sleep.

- The statement that "the tongue is the strongest muscle in the body" appears frequently in lists of surprising facts, but it is difficult to find any definition of "strength" that would make this statement true. Note that the tongue consists of eight muscles, not one.

- The heart has a claim to being the muscle that performs the largest quantity of physical work in the course of a lifetime. Estimates of the power output of the human heart range from 1 to 5 watts. This is much less than the maximum power output of other muscles; for example, the quadriceps can produce over 100 watts, but only for a few minutes. The heart does its work continuously over an entire lifetime without pause, and thus does "outwork" other muscles. An output of one watt continuously for eighty years yields a total work output of two and a half gigajoules.

Exercise

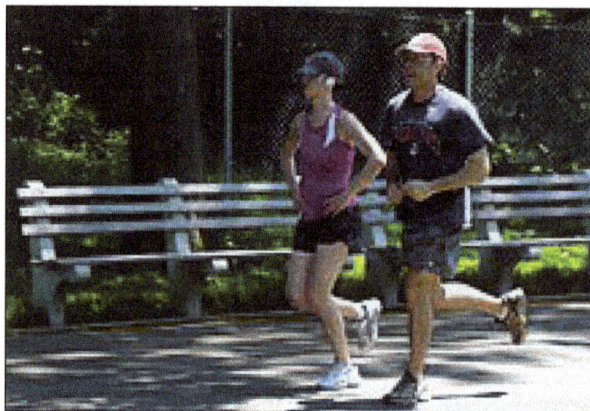

Jogging is one form of aerobic exercise.

Exercise is often recommended as a means of improving motor skills, fitness, muscle and bone strength, and joint function. Exercise has several effects upon muscles, connective tissue, bone, and the nerves that stimulate the muscles. One such effect is muscle hypertrophy, an increase in size. This is used in bodybuilding.

Various exercises require a predominance of certain muscle fiber utilization over another. Aerobic exercise involves long, low levels of exertion in which the muscles are used at well below their maximal contraction strength for long periods of time (the most classic example being the marathon). Aerobic events, which rely primarily on the aerobic (with oxygen) system, use a higher percentage of Type I (or slow-twitch) muscle fibers, consume a mixture of fat, protein and carbohydrates for energy, consume large amounts of oxygen and produce little lactic acid. Anaerobic exercise involves short bursts of higher intensity contractions at a much greater percentage of their maximum contraction strength. Examples of anaerobic exercise include sprinting and weight lifting. The anaerobic energy delivery system uses predominantly Type II or fast-twitch muscle fibers, relies mainly on ATP or glucose for fuel, consumes relatively little oxygen, protein and fat, produces large amounts of lactic acid and can not be sustained for as long a period as aerobic exercise. Many exercises are partially aerobic and partially anaerobic; for example, soccer and rock climbing involve a combination of both.

The presence of lactic acid has an inhibitory effect on ATP generation within the muscle; though not producing fatigue, it can inhibit or even stop performance if the intracellular concentration becomes too high. However, long-term training causes neovascularization within the muscle, increasing the ability to move waste products out of the muscles and maintain contraction. Once moved out of muscles with high concentrations within the sarcomere, lactic acid can be used by other muscles or body tissues as a source of energy, or transported to the liver where it is converted back to pyruvate. In addition to increasing the level of lactic acid, strenuous exercise causes the loss of potassium ions in muscle and causing an increase in potassium ion concentrations close to the muscle fibres, in the interstitium. Acidification by lactic acid may allow recovery of force so that acidosis may protect against fatigue rather than being a cause of fatigue.

Delayed onset muscle soreness is pain or discomfort that may be felt one to three days after exercising and generally subsides two to three days later. Once thought to be caused by lactic acid build-up, a more recent theory is that it is caused by tiny tears in the muscle fibers caused by eccentric contraction, or unaccustomed training levels. Since lactic acid disperses fairly rapidly, it could not explain pain experienced days after exercise.

CARTILAGE

Cartilage is a resilient and smooth elastic tissue, a rubber-like padding that covers and protects the ends of long bones at the joints, and is a structural component of the rib cage, the ear, the nose, the bronchial tubes, the intervertebral discs, and many other body components. It is not as hard and rigid as bone, but it is much stiffer and much less flexible than muscle. The matrix of cartilage is made up of glycosaminoglycans, proteoglycans, collagen fibers and, sometimes, elastin.

Because of its rigidity, cartilage often serves the purpose of holding tubes open in the body. Examples include the rings of the trachea, such as the cricoid cartilage and carina.

Cartilage is composed of specialized cells called chondrocytes that produce a large amount of collagenous extracellular matrix, abundant ground substance that is rich in proteoglycan and elastin fibers. Cartilage is classified in three types, *elastic cartilage*, *hyaline cartilage* and *fibrocartilage*, which differ in relative amounts of collagen and proteoglycan.

Cartilage does not contain blood vessels (it is avascular) or nerves (it is aneural). Nutrition is supplied to the chondrocytes by diffusion. The compression of the articular cartilage or flexion of the elastic cartilage generates fluid flow, which assists diffusion of nutrients to the chondrocytes. Compared to other connective tissues, cartilage has a very slow turnover of its extracellular matrix and does not repair.

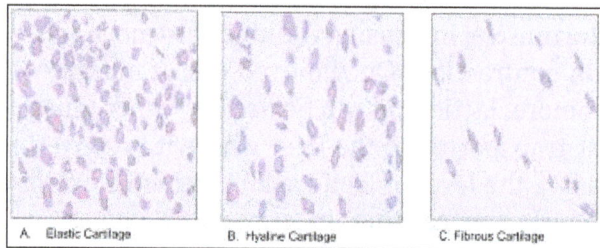

There are three different types of cartilage: elastic (A), hyaline (B), and fibrous (C). In elastic cartilage the cells are closer together creating less intercellular space.

Elastic cartilage is found in the external ear flaps and in parts of the larynx. Hyaline cartilage has fewer cells than elastic cartilage; there is more intercellular space. Hyaline cartilage is found in the nose, ears, trachea, parts of the larynx, and smaller respiratory tubes. Fibrous cartilage has the fewest cells so it has the most intercellular space. Fibrous cartilage is found in the spine and the menisci.

Structure

Development

In embryogenesis, the skeletal system is derived from the mesoderm germ layer. Chondrification (also known as chondrogenesis) is the process by which cartilage is formed from condensed mesenchyme tissue, which differentiates into chondroblasts and begins secreting the molecules (aggrecan and collagen type II) that form the extracellular matrix.

Following the initial chondrification that occurs during embryogenesis, cartilage growth consists mostly of the maturing of immature cartilage to a more mature state.

The division of cells within cartilage occurs very slowly, and thus growth in cartilage is usually not based on an increase in size or mass of the cartilage itself.

Articular Cartilage

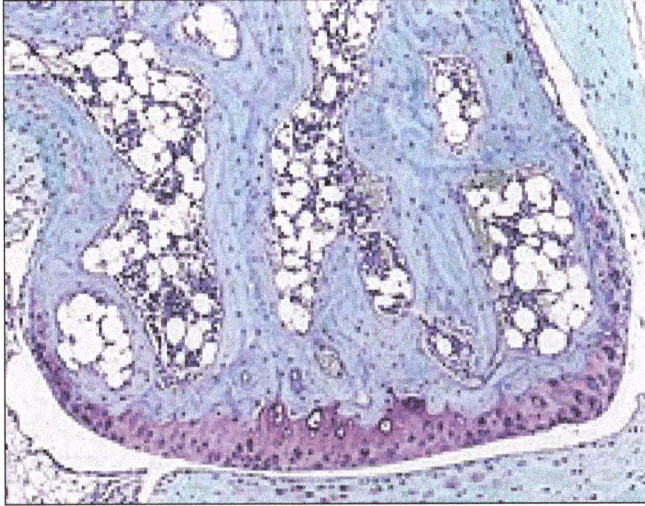

Mouse joint showing cartilage (purple).

The articular cartilage function is dependent on the molecular composition of the extracellular matrix (ECM). The ECM consists mainly of proteoglycan and collagens. The main proteoglycan in cartilage is aggrecan, which, as its name suggests, forms large aggregates with hyaluronan. These aggregates are negatively charged and hold water in the tissue. The collagen, mostly collagen type II, constrains the proteoglycans. The ECM responds to tensile and compressive forces that are experienced by the cartilage. Cartilage growth thus refers to the matrix deposition, but can also refer to both the growth and remodeling of the extracellular matrix. Due to the great stress on the patellofemoral joint during resisted knee extension, the articular cartilage of the patella is among the thickest in the human body.

Function

Mechanical Properties

The mechanical properties of articular cartilage in load-bearing joints such as the knee and hip have been studied extensively at macro, micro, and nano-scales. These mechanical properties include the response of cartilage in frictional, compressive, shear and tensile loading. Cartilage is resilient and displays viscoelastic properties.

Frictional Properties

Lubricin, a glycoprotein abundant in cartilage and synovial fluid, plays a major role in bio-lubrication and wear protection of cartilage.

Repair

Cartilage has limited repair capabilities: Because chondrocytes are bound in lacunae, they cannot migrate to damaged areas. Therefore, cartilage damage is difficult to heal. Also, because hyaline cartilage does not have a blood supply, the deposition of new matrix is slow. Damaged hyaline cartilage is usually replaced by fibrocartilage scar tissue. Over the last years, surgeons and scientists have elaborated a series of cartilage repair procedures that help to postpone the need for joint replacement.

Biological engineering techniques are being developed to generate new cartilage, using a cellular "scaffolding" material and cultured cells to grow artificial cartilage.

Clinical Significance

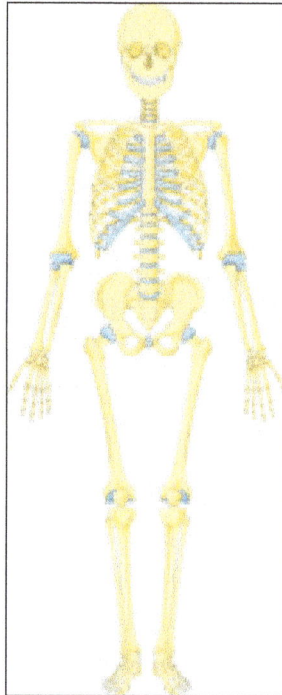

Human skeleton with articular cartilage shown in blue.

Disease

Several diseases can affect cartilage. Chondrodystrophies are a group of diseases, characterized by the disturbance of growth and subsequent ossification of cartilage. Some common diseases that affect the cartilage are listed below.

- Osteoarthritis: Osteoarthritis is a disease of the whole joint, however one of the most affected tissues is the articular cartilage. The cartilage covering bones (articular cartilage—a subset of hyaline cartilage) is thinned, eventually completely wearing away, resulting in a "bone against bone" within the joint, leading to reduced motion, and pain. Osteoarthritis affects the joints exposed to high stress and is therefore considered the result of "wear and tear" rather than a true disease. It is treated by arthroplasty, the replacement of the joint by a synthetic joint often made of a stainless steel alloy (cobalt chromoly) and ultra-high-molecular-weight polyethylene (UHMWPE). Chondroitin sulfate or glucosamine sulfate supplements, have been claimed to reduce the symptoms of osteoarthritis, but there is little good evidence to support this claim.

- Traumatic rupture or detachment: The cartilage in the knee is frequently damaged but can be partially repaired through knee cartilage replacement therapy. Often when athletes talk of damaged "cartilage" in their knee, they are referring to a damaged meniscus (a fibrocartilage structure) and not the articular cartilage.

- Achondroplasia: Reduced proliferation of chondrocytes in the epiphyseal plate of long bones during infancy and childhood, resulting in dwarfism.

- Costochondritis: Inflammation of cartilage in the ribs, causing chest pain.

- Spinal disc herniation: Asymmetrical compression of an intervertebral disc ruptures the sac-like disc, causing a herniation of its soft content. The hernia often compresses the adjacent nerves and causes back pain.

- Relapsing polychondritis: A destruction, probably autoimmune, of cartilage, especially of the nose and ears, causing disfiguration. Death occurs by asphyxiation as the larynx loses its rigidity and collapses.

Tumors made up of cartilage tissue, either benign or malignant, can occur. They usually appear in bone, rarely in pre-existing cartilage. The benign tumors are called chondroma, the malignant ones chondrosarcoma. Tumors arising from other tissues may also produce a cartilage-like matrix, the best known being pleomorphic adenoma of the salivary glands.

The matrix of cartilage acts as a barrier, preventing the entry of lymphocytes or diffusion of immunoglobulins. This property allows for the transplantation of cartilage from one individual to another without fear of tissue rejection.

Imaging

Cartilage does not absorb X-rays under normal *in vivo* conditions, but a dye can be injected into the synovial membrane that will cause the x-rays to be absorbed by the dye. The resulting void on the radiographic film between the bone and meniscus represents the cartilage. For In vitro x-ray scans, the outer soft tissue is most likely removed, so the cartilage and air boundary are enough to contrast the presence of cartilage due to the refraction of the x-ray.

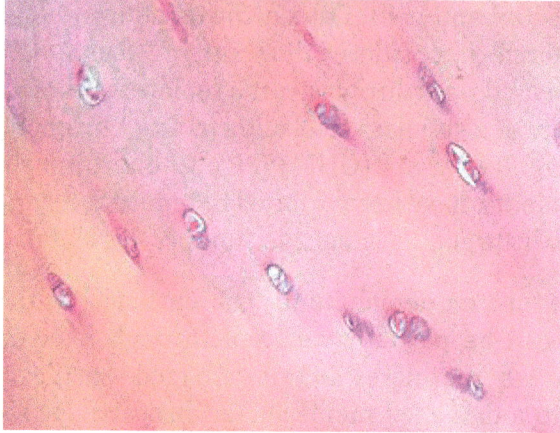

Histological image of hyaline cartilage stained with haematoxylin and eosin, under polarized light.

SKIN

Skin is the soft outer tissue covering of vertebrates with three main functions: protection, regulation, and sensation.

Other animal coverings, such as the arthropod exoskeleton, have different developmental origin, structure and chemical composition. The adjective cutaneous means "of the skin". In mammals, the skin is an organ of the integumentary system made up of multiple layers of ectodermal tissue, and guards the underlying muscles, bones, ligaments and internal organs. Skin of a different nature exists in amphibians, reptiles, and birds. All mammals have some hair on their skin, even marine mammals like whales, dolphins, and porpoises which appear to be hairless. The skin interfaces with the environment and is the first line of defense from external factors. For example, the skin plays a key role in protecting the body against pathogens and excessive water loss. Its other functions are insulation, temperature regulation, sensation, and the production of vitamin D folates. Severely damaged skin may heal by forming scar tissue. This is sometimes discoloured and depigmented. The thickness of skin also varies from location to location on an organism. In humans for example, the skin located under the eyes and around the eyelids is the thinnest skin in the body at 0.5 mm thick, and is one of the first areas to show signs of aging such as "crows feet" and wrinkles. The skin on the palms and the soles of the feet is 4 mm thick and is the thickest skin on the body. The speed and quality of wound healing in skin is promoted by the reception of estrogen.

Fur is dense hair. Primarily, fur augments the insulation the skin provides but can also serve as a secondary sexual characteristic or as camouflage. On some animals, the skin is very hard and thick, and can be processed to create leather. Reptiles and fish have hard protective scales on their skin for protection, and birds have hard feathers, all made of tough β-keratins. Amphibian skin is not a strong barrier, especially regarding the passage of chemicals via skin and is often subject to osmosis and diffusive forces. For example, a frog sitting in an anesthetic solution would be sedated quickly, as the chemical diffuses through its skin. Amphibian skin plays key roles in everyday survival and their ability to exploit a wide range of habitats and ecological conditions.

Structure in Humans and other Mammals

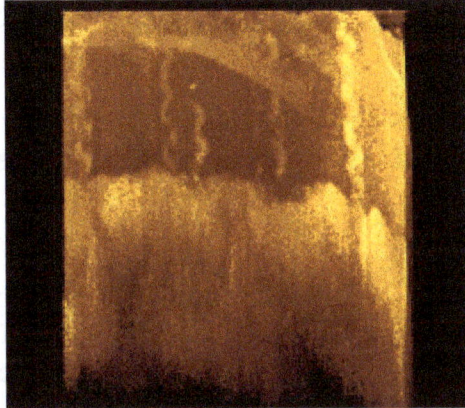

Optical coherence tomogram of fingertip, depicting stratum corneum (~500 μm thick) with stratum disjunctum on top and stratum lucidum (connection to stratum spinosum) in the middle. At the bottom superficial parts of the dermis. Sweatducts are clearly visible.

Mammalian skin is composed of two primary layers:

- The epidermis, which provides waterproofing and serves as a barrier to infection.

- The dermis, which serves as a location for the appendages of skin.

Epidermis

The epidermis is composed of the outermost layers of the skin. It forms a protective barrier over the body's surface, responsible for keeping water in the body and preventing pathogens from entering, and is a stratified squamous epithelium, composed of proliferating basal and differentiated suprabasal keratinocytes.

Keratinocytes are the major cells, constituting 95% of the epidermis, while Merkel cells, melanocytes and Langerhans cells are also present. The epidermis can be further subdivided into the following *strata* or layers (beginning with the outermost layer):

- Stratum corneum.

- Stratum lucidum (only in palms and soles).

- Stratum granulosum.

- Stratum spinosum.

- Stratum basale (also called the stratum germinativum).

Keratinocytes in the stratum basale proliferate through mitosis and the daughter cells move up the strata changing shape and composition as they undergo multiple stages of cell differentiation to eventually become anucleated. During that process, keratinocytes will become highly organized, forming cellular junctions (desmosomes) between each other and secreting keratin proteins and lipids which contribute to the formation of an extracellular matrix and provide mechanical strength to the skin. Keratinocytes from the stratum corneum are eventually shed from the surface (desquamation).

The epidermis contains no blood vessels, and cells in the deepest layers are nourished by diffusion from blood capillaries extending to the upper layers of the dermis.

Basement Membrane

The epidermis and dermis are separated by a thin sheet of fibers called the basement membrane, which is made through the action of both tissues. The basement membrane controls the traffic of the cells and molecules between the dermis and epidermis but also serves, through the binding of a variety of cytokines and growth factors, as a reservoir for their controlled release during physiological remodeling or repair processes.

Dermis

The dermis is the layer of skin beneath the epidermis that consists of connective tissue and cushions the body from stress and strain. The dermis provides tensile strength and elasticity to the skin through an extracellular matrix composed of collagen fibrils, microfibrils, and elastic fibers, embedded in hyaluronan and proteoglycans. Skin proteoglycans are varied and have very specific locations. For example, hyaluronan, versican and decorin are present throughout the dermis and epidermis extracellular matrix, whereas biglycan and perlecan are only found in the epidermis.

It harbors many mechanoreceptors (nerve endings) that provide the sense of touch and heat through nociceptors and thermoreceptors. It also contains the hair follicles, sweat glands, sebaceous glands, apocrine glands, lymphatic vessels and blood vessels. The blood vessels in the dermis provide nourishment and waste removal from its own cells as well as for the epidermis.

The dermis is tightly connected to the epidermis through a basement membrane and is structurally divided into two areas: a superficial area adjacent to the epidermis, called the *papillary region*, and a deep thicker area known as the *reticular region*.

Papillary Region

The papillary region is composed of loose areolar connective tissue. This is named for its fingerlike projections called *papillae* that extend toward the epidermis. The papillae provide the dermis with a "bumpy" surface that interdigitates with the epidermis, strengthening the connection between the two layers of skin.

Reticular Region

The reticular region lies deep in the papillary region and is usually much thicker. It is composed of dense irregular connective tissue and receives its name from the dense concentration of collagenous, elastic, and reticular fibers that weave throughout it. These protein fibers give the dermis its properties of strength, extensibility, and elasticity. Also located within the reticular region are the roots of the hair, sweat glands, sebaceous glands, receptors, nails, and blood vessels.

Subcutaneous Tissue

The subcutaneous tissue (also hypodermis) is not part of the skin, and lies below the dermis. Its purpose is to attach the skin to underlying bone and muscle as well as supplying it with blood vessels and nerves. It consists of loose connective tissue and elastin. The main cell types are fibroblasts, macrophages and adipocytes (the subcutaneous tissue contains 50% of body fat). Fat serves as padding and insulation for the body.

Microorganisms like *Staphylococcus epidermidis* colonize the skin surface. The density of skin flora depends on region of the skin. The disinfected skin surface gets recolonized from bacteria residing in the deeper areas of the hair follicle, gut and urogenital openings.

Cross Section

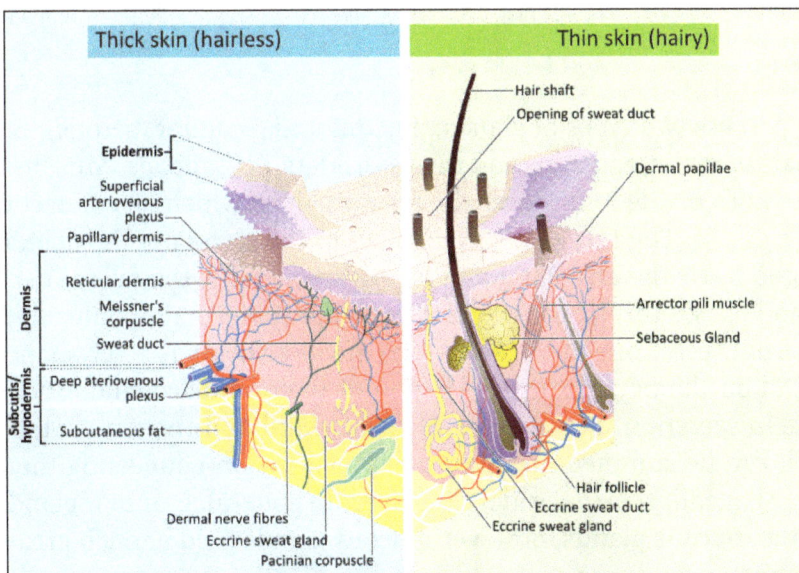

Skin layers, of both the hairy and hairless skin.

Structure in Fish, Amphibians, Birds and Reptiles

Fish

The epidermis of fish and of most amphibians consists entirely of live cells, with only minimal quantities of keratin in the cells of the superficial layer. It is generally permeable, and in the case of many amphibians, may actually be a major respiratory organ. The dermis of bony fish typically contains relatively little of the connective tissue found in tetrapods. Instead, in most species, it is largely replaced by solid, protective bony scales. Apart from some particularly large dermal bones that form parts of the skull, these scales are lost in tetrapods, although many reptiles do have scales of a different kind, as do pangolins. Cartilaginous fish have numerous tooth-like denticles embedded in their skin, in place of true scales.

Sweat glands and sebaceous glands are both unique to mammals, but other types of skin gland are found in other vertebrates. Fish typically have a numerous individual mucus-secreting skin cells that aid in insulation and protection, but may also have poison glands, photophores, or cells that produce a more watery, serous fluid. In amphibians, the mucus cells are gathered together to form sac-like glands. Most living amphibians also possess *granular glands* in the skin, that secrete irritating or toxic compounds.

Although melanin is found in the skin of many species, in the reptiles, the amphibians, and fish, the epidermis is often relatively colourless. Instead, the colour of the skin is largely due to chromatophores in the dermis, which, in addition to melanin, may contain guanine or carotenoid pigments. Many species, such as chameleons and flounders may be able to change the colour of their skin by adjusting the relative size of their chromatophores.

Amphibians

Amphibians possess two types of glands, mucous and granular (serous). Both of these glands are part of the integument and thus considered cutaneous. Mucous and granular glands are both divided into three different sections which all connect to structure the gland as a whole. The three individual parts of the gland are the duct, the intercalary region, and lastly the alveolar gland (sac). Structurally, the duct is derived via keratinocytes and passes through to the surface of the epidermal or outer skin layer thus allowing external secretions of the body. The gland alveolus is a sac shaped structure which is found on the bottom or base region of the granular gland. The cells in this sac specialize in secretion. Between the alveolar gland and the duct is the intercalary system which can be summed up as a transitional region connecting the duct to the grand alveolar beneath the epidermal skin layer. In general, granular glands are larger in size than the mucous glands, however mucous glands hold a much greater majority in overall number.

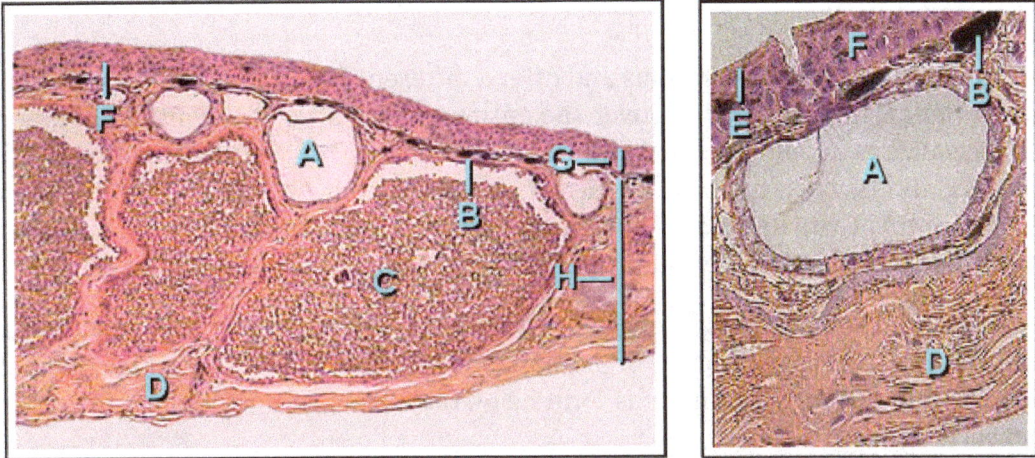

Frog Gland Anatomy- A: Mucous gland (alveolus), B: Chromophore, C: Granular Gland (alveolus), D: Connective Tissue, E: Stratum Corneum, F: Transition Zone (intercalary region), G: Epidermis (Where the duct resides), H: Dermis.

Granular Glands

Granular glands can be identified as venomous and often differ in the type of toxin as well as the concentrations of secretions across various orders and species within the amphibians. They are located in clusters differing in concentration depending on amphibian taxa. The toxins can be fatal to most vertebrates or have no effect against others. These glands are alveolar meaning they structurally have little sacs in which venom is produced and held before it is secreted upon defensive behaviors.

Structurally, the ducts of the granular gland initially maintain a cylindrical shape. However, when the ducts become mature and full of toxic fluid, the base of the ducts become swollen due to the pressure from the inside. This causes the epidermal layer to form a pit like opening on the surface of the duct in which the inner fluid will be secreted in an upwards fashion.

The intercalary region of granular glands are more developed and mature in comparison with mucous glands. This region resides as a ring of cells surrounding the basal portion of the duct which are argued to have an ectodermal muscular nature due to their influence over the lumen (space inside the tube) of the duct with dilation and constriction functions during secretions. The cells are found radially around the duct and provide a distinct attachment site for muscle fibers around the gland's body.

The gland alveolus is a sac that is divided into three specific regions/layers. The outer layer or tunica fibrosa is composed of densely packed connective-tissue which connects with fibers from the spongy intermediate layer where elastic fibers as well as nerves reside. The nerves send signals to the muscles as well as the epithelial layers. Lastly, the epithelium or tunica propria encloses the gland.

Mucous Glands

Mucous glands are non-venomous and offer a different functionality for amphibians than granular. Mucous glands cover the entire surface area of the amphibian body and specialize in keeping the body lubricated. There are many other functions of the mucous glands such as controlling the pH, thermoregulation, adhesive properties to the environment, anti-predator behaviors (slimy to the grasp), chemical communication, even anti-bacterial/viral properties for protection against pathogens.

The ducts of the mucous gland appear as cylindrical vertical tubes which break through the epidermal layer to the surface of the skin. The cells lining the inside of the ducts are oriented with their longitudinal axis forming 90 degree angles surrounding the duct in a helical fashion.

Intercalary cells react identically to those of granular glands but on a smaller scale. Among the amphibians, there are taxa which contain a modified intercalary region (depending on the function of the glands), yet the majority share the same structure.

The alveolor of mucous glands are much more simple and only consist of an epithelium layer as well as connective tissue which forms a cover over the gland. This gland lacks a tunica propria and appears to have delicate and intricate fibers which pass over the gland's muscle and epithelial layers.

Birds and Reptiles

The epidermis of birds and reptiles is closer to that of mammals, with a layer of dead keratin-filled cells at the surface, to help reduce water loss. A similar pattern is also seen in some of the more terrestrial amphibians such as toads. However, in all of these animals there is no clear differentiation of the epidermis into distinct layers, as occurs in humans, with the change in cell type being relatively gradual. The mammalian epidermis always possesses at least a stratum germinativum and stratum corneum, but the other intermediate layers found in humans are not always distinguishable. Hair is a distinctive feature of mammalian skin, while feathers are (at least among living species) similarly unique to birds.

Birds and reptiles have relatively few skin glands, although there may be a few structures for specific purposes, such as pheromone-secreting cells in some reptiles, or the uropygial gland of most birds.

Development

Cutaneous structures arise from the epidermis and include a variety of features such as hair, feathers, claws and nails. During embryogenesis, the epidermis splits into two layers: the periderm (which is lost) and the basal layer. The basal layer is a stem cell layer and through asymmetrical divisions, becomes the source of skin cells throughout life.

It is maintained as a stem cell layer through an autocrine signal, TGF-a, and through paracrine signal FGF7 aka keratinocyte growth factor (KGF) produced by the dermis below the basal cells. In mice, over-expression of these factors leads to an overproduction of granule cells and thick skin.

Hair and feathers are formed in a regular pattern and it is believed to be the result of a reaction-diffusion system. This reaction-diffusion system combines an activator, Sonic hedgehog, with an inhibitor, BMP4 or BMP2, to form clusters of cells in a regular pattern. Sonic hedgehog-expressing epidermal cells induce the condensation of cells in the mesoderm. The clusters of mesodermal cells signal back to the epidermis to form the appropriate structure for that position. BMP signals from the epidermis inhibit the formation of placodes in nearby ectoderm.

It is believed that the mesoderm defines the pattern. The epidermis instructs the mesodermal cells to condense and then the mesoderm instructs the epidermis of what structure to make through a series of reciprocal inductions. Transplantation experiments involving frog and newt epidermis indicated that the mesodermal signals are conserved between species but the epidermal response is species-specific meaning that the mesoderm instructs the epidermis of its position and the epidermis uses this information to make a specific structure.

Functions

Skin performs the following functions:

- Protection: An anatomical barrier from pathogens and damage between the internal and external environment in bodily defense. Langerhans cells in the skin are part of the adaptive immune system.

- Sensation: Contains a variety of nerve endings that jump to heat and cold, touch, pressure, vibration, and tissue injury.

- Thermoregulation: Eccrine (sweat) glands and dilated blood vessels (increased superficial perfusion) aid heat loss, while constricted vessels greatly reduce cutaneous blood flow and conserve heat. Erector pili muscles in mammals adjust the angle of hair shafts to change the degree of insulation provided by hair or fur.

- Control of evaporation: The skin provides a relatively dry and semi-impermeable barrier to reduce fluid loss.

- Storage and synthesis: Acts as a storage center for lipids and water.

- Absorption through the skin: Oxygen, nitrogen and carbon dioxide can diffuse into the epidermis in small amounts; some animals use their skin as their sole respiration organ (in humans, the cells comprising the outermost 0.25–0.40 mm of the skin are "almost exclusively supplied by external oxygen", although the "contribution to total respiration is negligible") Some medications are absorbed through the skin.

- Water resistance: The skin acts as a water resistant barrier so essential nutrients aren't washed out of the body. The nutrients and oils that help hydrate the skin are covered by the most outer skin layer, the epidermis. This is helped in part by the sebaceous glands that release sebum, an oily liquid. Water itself will not cause the elimination of oils on the skin, because the oils residing in our dermis flow and would be affected by water without the epidermis.

- Camouflage: Whether the skin is naked or covered in fur, scales, or feathers, skin structures provide protective coloration and patterns that help to conceal animals from predators or prey.

Mechanics

Skin is a soft tissue and exhibits key mechanical behaviors of these tissues. The most pronounced feature is the J-curve stress strain response, in which a region of large strain and minimal stress exists and corresponds to the microstructural straightening and reorientation of collagen fibrils. In some cases the intact skin is prestreched, like wetsuits around the diver's body, and in other cases the intact skin is under compression. Small circular holes punched on the skin may widen or close into ellipses, or shrink and remain circular, depending on preexisting stresses.

Aging

Tissue homeostasis generally declines with age, in part because stem/progenitor cells fail to self-renew or differentiate. In the skin of mice, mitochondrial oxidative stress can promote cellular senescence and aging phenotypes. Ordinarily mitochondrial superoxide dismutase (SOD_2) protects against oxidative stress. Using a mouse model of genetic SOD2 deficiency, it was shown that failure to express this important antioxidant enzyme in epidermal cells caused cellular senescence, nuclear DNA damage, and irreversible arrest of proliferation of a fraction of keratinocytes.

Skin aging is caused in part by TGF-β, which reduces the subcutaneous fat that gives skin a pleasant appearance and texture. TGF-β does this by blocking the conversion of dermal fibroblasts into fat cells; with fewer fat cells underneath to provide support, the skin becomes saggy and wrinkled. Subcutaneous fat also produces cathelicidin, which is a peptide that fights bacterial infections.

TENDON

A tendon or sinew is a tough band of fibrous connective tissue that connects muscle to bone and is capable of withstanding tension.

Tendons are similar to ligaments; both are made of collagen. Ligaments connect one bone to another, while tendons connect muscle to bone.

Structure

Histologically, tendons consist of dense regular connective tissue. The main cellular component of tendons are specialized fibroblasts called the tenocytes. Tenocytes synthesize the extracellular matrix of tendons, abundant in densely packed collagen fibers. The collagen fibers are parallel to each other and organized into fascicles. Individual fascicles are bound by the endotendineum, which is a delicate loose connective tissue containing thin collagen fibrils and elastic fibres. Groups of fascicles are bounded by the epitenon, which are the sheaths of dense irregular connective tissue. The whole tendon is enclosed by a fascia. The space between the facsia and the tendon tissue is filled with the paratenon, a fatty areolar tissue. Normal healthy tendons are anchored to bone by Sharpey's fibres.

Extracellular Matrix

The dry mass of normal tendons, which makes up about 30% of their total mass, is composed of:

- Around 86% collagen.

- 2% elastin.

- 1–5% proteoglycans.

- 0.2% inorganic components such as copper, manganese, and calcium.

The collagen portion is made up of 97–98% type I collagen, with small amounts of other types of collagen. These include type II collagen in the cartilaginous zones, type III collagen in the reticulin fibres of the vascular walls, type IX collagen, type IV collagen in the basement membranes of the capillaries, type V collagen in the vascular walls, and type X collagen in the mineralized fibrocartilage near the interface with the bone.

Ultrastructure and Collagen Synthesis

Collagen fibres coalesce into macroaggregates. After secretion from the cell, cleaved by procollagen N- and C-proteinases, the tropocollagen molecules spontaneously assemble into insoluble fibrils. A collagen molecule is about 300 nm long and 1–2 nm wide, and the diameter of the fibrils that are formed can range from 50–500 nm. In tendons, the fibrils then assemble further to form fascicles, which are about 10 mm in length with a diameter of 50–300 µm, and finally into a tendon fibre with a diameter of 100–500 µm.

The collagen in tendons are held together with proteoglycan (a compound consisting of a protein bonded to glycosaminoglycan groups, present especially in connective tissue) components including decorin and, in compressed regions of tendon, aggrecan, which are capable of binding to the collagen fibrils at specific locations. The proteoglycans are interwoven with the collagen fibrils – their glycosaminoglycan (GAG) side chains have multiple interactions with the surface of the fibrils – showing that the proteoglycans are important structurally in the interconnection of the fibrils. The major GAG components of the tendon are dermatan sulfate and chondroitin sulfate, which associate with collagen and are involved in the fibril assembly process during tendon development. Dermatan sulfate is thought to be responsible for forming associations between fibrils, while chondroitin sulfate is thought to be more involved with occupying volume between the fibrils to keep them separated and help withstand deformation. The dermatan sulfate side chains of decorin aggregate in solution, and this behavior can assist with the assembly of the collagen fibrils. When decorin molecules are bound to a collagen fibril, their dermatan sulfate chains may extend and associate with other dermatan sulfate chains on decorin that is bound to separate fibrils, therefore creating interfibrillar bridges and eventually causing parallel alignment of the fibrils.

Tenocytes

The tenocytes produce the collagen molecules, which aggregate end-to-end and side-to-side to produce collagen fibrils. Fibril bundles are organized to form fibres with the elongated tenocytes closely packed between them. There is a three-dimensional network of cell processes associated with collagen in the tendon. The cells communicate with each other through gap junctions, and this signalling gives them the ability to detect and respond to mechanical loading.

Blood vessels may be visualized within the endotendon running parallel to collagen fibres, with occasional branching transverse anastomoses.

The internal tendon bulk is thought to contain no nerve fibres, but the epitenon and paratenon contain nerve endings, while Golgi tendon organs are present at the junction between tendon and muscle.

Tendon length varies in all major groups and from person to person. Tendon length is, in practice, the deciding factor regarding actual and potential muscle size. For example, all other relevant biological factors being equal, a man with a shorter tendons and a longer biceps muscle will have greater potential for muscle mass than a man with a longer tendon and a shorter muscle. Successful bodybuilders will generally have shorter tendons. Conversely, in sports requiring athletes to excel in actions such as running or jumping, it is beneficial to have longer than average Achilles tendon and a shorter calf muscle.

Tendon length is determined by genetic predisposition, and has not been shown to either increase or decrease in response to environment, unlike muscles, which can be shortened by trauma, use imbalances and a lack of recovery and stretching.

Functions

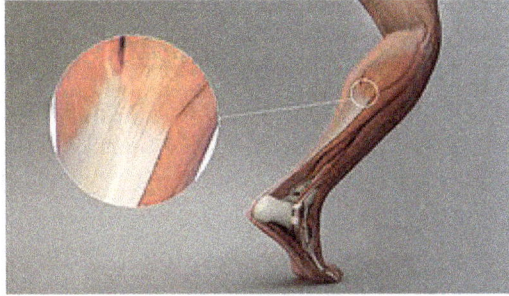

Magnified view of a tendon.

Traditionally, tendons have been considered to be a mechanism by which muscles connect to bone as well as muscles itself, functioning to transmit forces. This connection allows tendons to passively modulate forces during locomotion, providing additional stability with no active work. However, over the past two decades, much research focused on the elastic properties of some tendons and their ability to function as springs. Not all tendons are required to perform the same functional role, with some predominantly positioning limbs, such as the fingers when writing (positional tendons) and others acting as springs to make locomotion more efficient (energy storing tendons). Energy storing tendons can store and recover energy at high efficiency. For example, during a human stride, the Achilles tendon stretches as the ankle joint dorsiflexes. During the last portion of the stride, as the foot plantar-flexes (pointing the toes down), the stored elastic energy is released. Furthermore, because the tendon stretches, the muscle is able to function with less or even no change in length, allowing the muscle to generate greater force.

The mechanical properties of the tendon are dependent on the collagen fiber diameter and orientation. The collagen fibrils are parallel to each other and closely packed, but show a wave-like appearance due to planar undulations, or crimps, on a scale of several micrometers. In tendons, the collagen fibres have some flexibility due to the absence of hydroxyproline and proline residues at specific locations in the amino acid sequence, which allows the formation of other conformations such as bends or internal loops in the triple helix and results in the development of crimps. The crimps in the collagen fibrils allow the tendons to have some flexibility as well as a low compressive stiffness. In addition, because the tendon is a multi-stranded structure made up of many partially independent fibrils and fascicles, it does not behave as a single rod, and this property also contributes to its flexibility.

The proteoglycan components of tendons also are important to the mechanical properties. While the collagen fibrils allow tendons to resist tensile stress, the proteoglycans allow them to resist compressive stress. These molecules are very hydrophilic, meaning that they can absorb a large amount of water and therefore have a high swelling ratio. Since they are noncovalently bound to the fibrils, they may reversibly associate and disassociate so that the bridges between fibrils can be broken and reformed. This process may be involved in allowing the fibril to elongate and decrease in diameter under tension. However, the proteoglycans may also have a role in the tensile properties of tendon. The structure of tendon is effectively a fibre composite material, built as a series of hierarchical levels. At each level of the hierarchy, the collagen units are bound together by either collagen crosslinks, or the proteoglycans, to create a structure highly resistant to tensile load. The elongation and the strain of the collagen fibrils alone have been shown to be much lower than the total elongation and strain of the entire tendon under the same amount of stress, demonstrating that the proteoglycan-rich matrix must also undergo deformation, and stiffening of the matrix occurs at high strain rates. This deformation of the non-collagenous matrix occurs at all levels of the tendon hierarchy, and by modulating the organisation and structure of this matrix, the different mechanical properties required by different tendons can be achieved. Energy storing tendons have been shown to utilise significant amounts of sliding between fascicles to enable the high strain characteristics they require, whilst positional tendons rely more heavily on sliding between collagen fibres and fibrils. However, recent data suggests that energy storing tendons may also contain fascicles which are twisted, or helical, in nature - an arrangement that would be highly beneficial for providing the spring-like behaviour required in these tendons.

Mechanics

Tendons are viscoelastic structures, which means they exhibit both elastic and viscous behaviour. When stretched, tendons exhibit typical "soft tissue" behavior. The force-extension, or stress-strain curve starts with a very low stiffness region, as the crimp structure straightens and the collagen fibres align suggesting negative Poisson's ratio in the fibres of the tendon. More recently, tests carried out in vivo (through MRI) and ex vivo (through mechanical testing of various cadaveric tendon tissue) have shown that healthy tendons are highly anisotropic and exhibit a negative Poisson's ratio (auxetic) in some planes when stretched up to 2% along their length, i.e. within their normal range of motion. After this 'toe' region, the structure becomes significantly stiffer, and has a linear stress-strain curve until it begins to fail. The mechanical properties of tendons vary widely, as they are matched to the functional requirements of the tendon. The energy storing tendons tend to be more elastic, or less stiff, so they can more easily store energy, whilst the stiffer positional tendons tend to be a little more viscoelastic, and less elastic, so they can provide finer control of movement. A typical energy storing tendon will fail at around 12-15% strain, and a stress in the region of 100-150 MPa, although some tendons are notably more extensible than this, for example the superficial digital flexor in the horse, which stretches in excess of 20% when galloping. Positional tendons can fail at strains as low as 6-8%, but can have moduli in the region of 700-1000 MPa.

Several studies have demonstrated that tendons respond to changes in mechanical loading with growth and remodeling processes, much like bones. In particular, a study showed that disuse of the Achilles tendon in rats resulted in a decrease in the average thickness of the collagen fiber bundles comprising the tendon. In humans, an experiment in which people were subjected to a simulated micro-gravity environment found that tendon stiffness decreased significantly, even when subjects were required to perform restiveness exercises. These effects have implications in areas ranging from treatment of bedridden patients to the design of more effective exercises for astronauts.

Healing

The tendons in the foot are highly complex and intricate. Therefore, the healing process for a broken tendon is long and painful. Most people who do not receive medical attention within the first 48 hours of the injury will suffer from severe swelling, pain, and a burning sensation where the injury occurred.

It was believed that tendons could not undergo matrix turnover and that tenocytes were not capable of repair. However, it has since been shown that, throughout the lifetime of a person, tenocytes in the tendon actively synthesize matrix components as well as enzymes such as matrix metalloproteinases (MMPs) can degrade the matrix. Tendons are capable of healing and recovering from injuries in a process that is controlled by the tenocytes and their surrounding extracellular matrix.

The three main stages of tendon healing are inflammation, repair or proliferation, and remodeling, which can be further divided into consolidation and maturation. These stages can overlap with each other. In the first stage, inflammatory cells such as neutrophils are recruited to the injury site, along with erythrocytes. Monocytes and macrophages are recruited within the first 24 hours, and phagocytosis of necrotic materials at the injury site occurs. After the release of vasoactive and chemotactic factors, angiogenesis and the proliferation of tenocytes are initiated. Tenocytes then move into the site and start to synthesize collagen III. After a few days, the repair or proliferation stage begins. In this stage, the tenocytes are involved in the synthesis of large amounts of collagen and proteoglycans at the site of injury, and the levels of GAG and water are high. After about six weeks, the remodeling stage begins. The first part of this stage is consolidation, which lasts from about six to ten weeks after the injury. During this time, the synthesis of collagen and GAGs is decreased, and the cellularity is also decreased as the tissue becomes more fibrous as a result of increased production of collagen I and the fibrils become aligned in the direction of mechanical stress. The final maturation stage occurs after ten weeks, and during this time there is an increase in crosslinking of the collagen fibrils, which causes the tissue to become stiffer. Gradually, over about one year, the tissue will turn from fibrous to scar-like.

Matrix metalloproteinases (MMPs) have a very important role in the degradation and remodeling of the ECM during the healing process after a tendon injury. Certain MMPs including MMP-1, MMP-2, MMP-8, MMP-13, and MMP-14 have collagenase activity, meaning that, unlike many other enzymes, they are capable of degrading collagen I fibrils. The degradation of the collagen fibrils by MMP-1 along with the presence of denatured collagen are factors that are believed to cause weakening of the tendon ECM and an increase in the potential for another rupture to occur. In response to repeated mechanical loading or injury, cytokines may be released by tenocytes and can induce the release of MMPs, causing degradation of the ECM and leading to recurring injury and chronic tendinopathies.

A variety of other molecules are involved in tendon repair and regeneration. There are five growth factors that have been shown to be significantly upregulated and active during tendon healing: insulin-like growth factor 1 (IGF-I), platelet-derived growth factor (PDGF), vascular endothelial growth factor (VEGF), basic fibroblast growth factor (bFGF), and transforming growth factor beta (TGF-β). These growth factors all have different roles during the healing process. IGF-1 increases collagen and proteoglycan production during the first stage of inflammation, and PDGF is also present during the early stages after injury and promotes the synthesis of other growth factors along with the synthesis of DNA and the proliferation of tendon cells. The three isoforms of TGF-β (TGF-β1, TGF-β2, TGF-β3) are known to play a role in wound healing and scar formation. VEGF is well known to promote angiogenesis and to induce endothelial cell proliferation and migration, and VEGF mRNA has been shown to be expressed at the site of tendon injuries along with collagen I mRNA. Bone morphogenetic proteins (BMPs) are a subgroup of TGF-β superfamily that can induce bone and cartilage formation as well as tissue differentiation, and BMP-12 specifically has been shown to influence formation and differentiation of tendon tissue and to promote fibrogenesis.

Effects of Activity on Healing

In animal models, extensive studies have been conducted to investigate the effects of mechanical strain in the form of activity level on tendon injury and healing. While stretching can disrupt healing during the initial inflammatory phase, it has been shown that controlled movement of the tendons after about one week following an acute injury can help to promote the synthesis of collagen by the tenocytes, leading to increased tensile strength and diameter of the healed tendons and fewer adhesions than tendons that are immobilized. In chronic tendon injuries, mechanical loading has also been shown to stimulate fibroblast proliferation and collagen synthesis along with collagen realignment, all of which promote repair and remodeling. To further support the theory that movement and activity assist in tendon healing, it has been shown that immobilization of the tendons after injury often has a negative effect on healing. In rabbits, collagen fascicles that are immobilized have shown decreased tensile strength, and immobilization also results in lower amounts of water, proteoglycans, and collagen crosslinks in the tendons.

Several mechanotransduction mechanisms have been proposed as reasons for the response of tenocytes to mechanical force that enable them to alter their gene expression, protein synthesis, and cell phenotype, and eventually cause changes in tendon structure. A major factor is mechanical deformation of the extracellular matrix, which can affect the actin cytoskeleton and therefore affect cell shape, motility, and function. Mechanical forces can be transmitted by focal adhesion sites, integrins, and cell-cell junctions. Changes in the actin cytoskeleton can activate integrins, which mediate "outside-in" and "inside-out" signaling between the cell and the matrix. G-proteins, which induce intracellular signaling cascades, may also be important, and ion channels are activated by stretching to allow ions such as calcium, sodium, or potassium to enter the cell.

Clinical Significance

Injury

Tendons are subject to many types of injuries. There are various forms of tendinopathies or tendon injuries due to overuse. These types of injuries generally result in inflammation and degeneration or weakening of the tendons, which may eventually lead to tendon rupture. Tendinopathies can be caused by a number of factors relating to the tendon extracellular matrix (ECM), and their classification has been difficult because their symptoms and histopathology often are similar.

The first category of tendinopathy is paratenonitis, which refers to inflammation of the paratenon, or paratendinous sheet located between the tendon and its sheath. Tendinosis refers to non-inflammatory injury to the tendon at the cellular level. The degradation is caused by damage to collagen, cells, and the vascular components of the tendon, and is known to lead to rupture. Observations of tendons that have undergone spontaneous rupture have shown the presence of collagen fibrils that are not in the correct parallel orientation or are not uniform in length or diameter, along with rounded tenocytes, other cell abnormalities, and the ingrowth of blood vessels. Other forms of tendinosis that have not led to rupture have also shown the degeneration, disorientation, and thinning of the collagen fibrils, along with an increase in the amount of glycosaminoglycans between the fibrils. The third is paratenonitis with tendinosis, in which combinations of paratenon inflammation and tendon degeneration are both present. The last is tendinitis, which refers to degeneration with inflammation of the tendon as well as vascular disruption.

Tendinopathies may be caused by several intrinsic factors including age, body weight, and nutrition. The extrinsic factors are often related to sports and include excessive forces or loading, poor training techniques, and environmental conditions.

Tendon Structure and Composition

Tendons have a hierarchical arrangement that is sequentially composed of collagen molecules, fibrils, fibres, fascicles, and lastly the tendon unit. Tendon units are encased in epitenon, which reduces friction with neighbouring tissues.

The tensile strength of a tendon is dependent on collagen. Type I collagen comprises approximately 70–80% of the dry weight of a normal tendon. Additional to type I collagen, many other types of collagen are also present, including type III (functions to form rapid cross-links in stabilizing repair sites in torn tendons), type V (regulates collagen fibril diameter), and type XII (provides lubrication between collagen fibres).

In addition to collagen, many proteoglycans (e.g. aggrecan and decorin) and glycoproteins (e.g. elastin, fibronectin, and tenascin-C) also have important functions in tendons. Aggrecan binds water and resists compression, while decorin promotes fibrillar slippage. Elastin, fibronectin, and tenascin-C function to enhance mechanical stability, aid tendon healing, and allow tendons to revert back to their pre-stretched lengths after normal physiological loading, respectively.

Tendon Mechanical Properties: Non-linear Elasticity

The structure and composition of tendons allow for their unique mechanical behavior, reflected by a stress-strain curve consisting of three distinct regions:

- Toe region: This is where "stretching out" or "un-crimping" of crimped tendon fibrils occurs from mechanically loading the tendon up to 2% strain. This region is responsible for nonlinear stress/strain curve, because the slope of the toe region is not linear.

- Linear region: This is the physiological upper limit of tendon strain whereby the collagen fibrils orient themselves in the direction of tensile mechanical load and begin to stretch. The tendon deforms in a linear fashion due to the inter-molecular sliding of collagen triple helices. If strain is less than 4%, the tendon will return to its original length when unloaded, therefore this portion is elastic and reversible and the slope of the curve represents the Young's modulus.

- Yield and failure region: This is where the tendon stretches beyond its physiological limit and intramolecular cross-links between collagen fibres fail. If micro-failure continues to accumulate, stiffness is reduced and the tendon begins to fail, resulting in irreversible plastic deformation. If the tendon stretches beyond 8-10% of its original length, macroscopic failure soon follows.

Since there are many muscles in the body, each tendon differs in its function and therefore its mechanical properties. For example, the Young's modulus of the human patellar tendon is 660 ± 266 MPa (mean ± standard deviation),whereas the tibialis anterior tendon is about 1200 MPa. Aging also significantly affects the mechanical properties of tendons:Young's modulus of human patellar tendons aged 29–50 years is about 660 ± 266 MPa, but is about 504 ± 222 MPa in those aged 64–93 years.

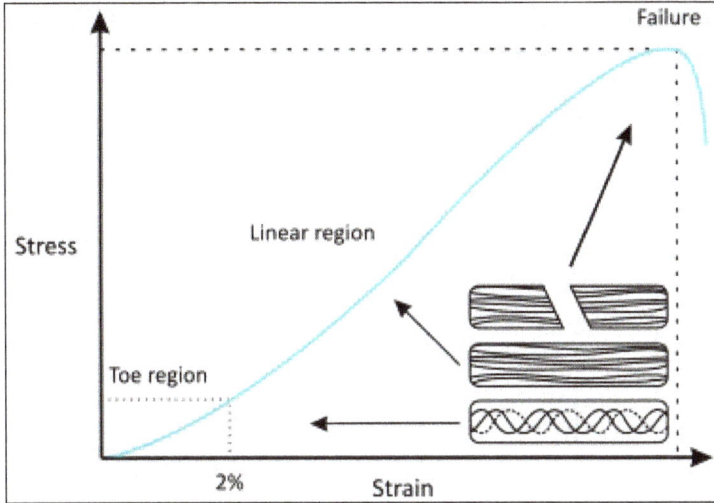

Tendon Mechanical Properties: Viscoelasticity

Tendons also have viscoelastic properties (likely the result of collagenous proteins, water, and the interactions between collagens and proteoglycans), meaning their mechanical behaviour is dependent on the rate of mechanical strain. In other words, the relationship between stress and strain for a tendon is not constant but depends on the time of displacement or load. A viscoeleastic material is more deformable at low strain rates but less deformable at high strain rates. Therefore, tendons at low strain rates tend to absorb more mechanical energy but are less effective in carrying mechanical loads. However, tendons become stiffer and more effective in transmitting large muscular loads to bone at high strain rates.

There are three major characteristics of a viscoelastic material of tendons.

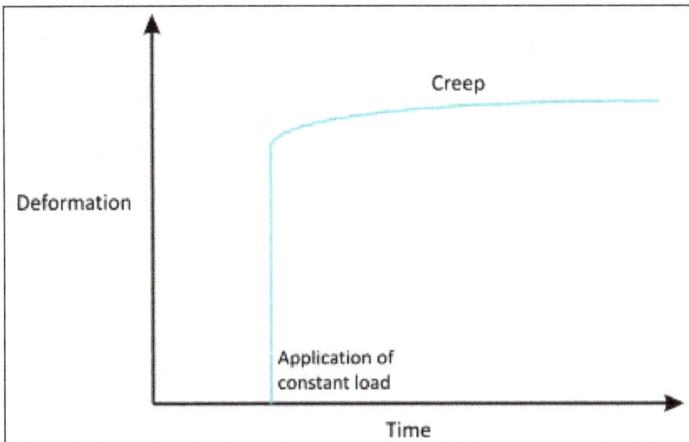

Creep:

- Indicates increasing deformation under constant load.

- This is in contrast with the usual elastic material, which does not elongate, no matter how long the load is applied.

Stress relaxation:

- Indicates stress acting upon a tendon will eventually reduce under a constant deformation.

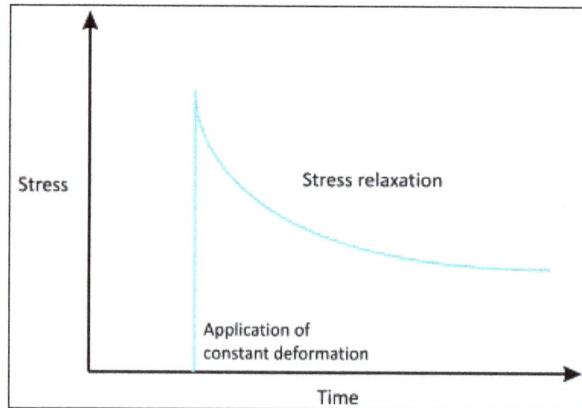

Hysteresis or energy dissipation:

- When a viscoelastic material is loaded and unloaded, the unloading curve is different from the loading curve.

- The difference between the two curves represents the amount of energy that is lost during loading.

- If loading and unloading are repeated several times, different curves can be obtained.

- After about 10 cycles, however, the loading and unloading curves no longer change (although they are still different) and the amount of hysteresis is reduced allowing the stress-strain curve to become reproducible.

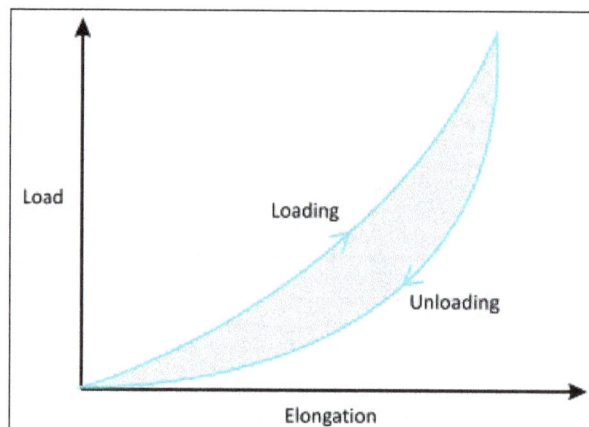

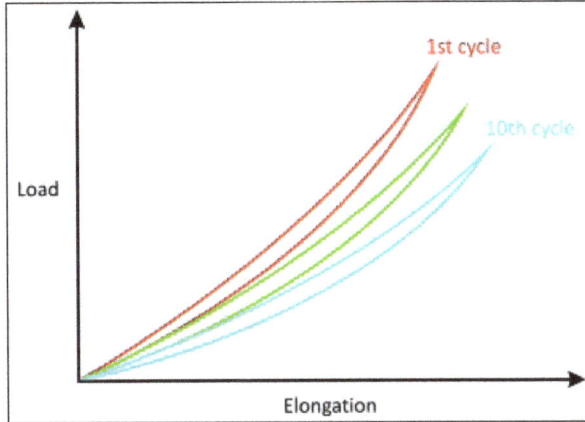

Factors Affecting Mechanical Forces

Many factors affect the mechanical forces on tendons during normal locomotion.

First, different tendons in the body are subjected to different levels of mechanical loads. For example, it has been estimated that the peak force transmitted through the Achilles tendon in humans during running is 9 kN, which is equivalent to 12.5 times body weight.In human hand flexor tendons, it has been shown that the intratendinous force of the tendon depends on whether the force is generated passively or actively, and whether the position of the joint is in flexion or extension. During passive mobilization of the wrist, the flexor tendon force was found to be between 1-6 N and up to 9 N during similar mobilization of the fingers. During a 35 N fingertip pinch, tendon forces can be measured up to 12 N whereas during active, unresisted finger motion, tendon force can reach approximately 35 N.

Second, both the level of muscle contraction and the tendon's relative size influence mechanical forces on a tendon. In general, the greater the cross-sectional area of a muscle, the higher force it can produce and the larger stress its tendon undergoes (e.g. patellar tendon vs. hamstring).

Third, different activities induce different levels of forces, even on the same tendon (in animal models).Similarly, varying the rate and frequency of mechanical loading results in different tendon forces.

The Differential Effects of Mechanical Loading on Tendons

Mechanical Load Level	Effects on Tendon
Low	• ↓ Tensile strength. • ↓ Size. • ↓ Collagen production. • ↓ Anabolic activities. • ↑ Catabolic activities.

Moderate	• ↑ Tensile strength. • ↑ Collagen synthesis. • ↓ Collagen degradation. • ↓ Adhesions. • ↓ Inflammatory mediator (e.g. prostaglandin E2). • ↑ Tendon stem cells (TSCs) differentiating into tenocytes.
Excessive	• ↓ Tensile strength. • ↓ Collagen organization. • ↑ Myofibroblasts. • ↑ Inflammatory mediators. • ↑ TSCs differentiating into nontenocytes (adipocytes, osteocytes, chondrocytes). • ↑ Leukotrienes (↑ edema).

Normal tendons can show a disorganised response to loading as well as improved tendon structure with over long term loading.

References

- Biological-hard-tissue, engineering: sciencedirect.com, Retrieved 05 April, 2019

- Mohamed, Amar; Alkhaledi, K.; Cochran, D. (2014). "Estimation of mechanical properties of soft tissue subjected to dynamic impact". Journal of Engineering Research. 2 (4): 87–101. doi:10.7603/s40632-014-0026-8

- MacIntosh, BR; Gardiner, PF; McComas, AJ (2006). "1. Muscle Architecture and Muscle Fiber Anatomy". Skeletal Muscle: Form and Function (2nd ed.). Champaign, IL: Human Kinetics. pp. 3–21. ISBN 978-0-7360-4517-9

- Asanbaeva A, Masuda K, Thonar EJ, Klisch SM, Sah RL (2008). "Cartilage growth and remodeling: Modulation of balance between proteoglycan and collagen network in vitro with β-aminopropionitrile1". Osteoarthritis and Cartilage. 16 (1): 1–11. doi:10.1016/j.joca.2007.05.019

- Tendon-Biomechanics: physio-pedia.com, Retrieved 29 August, 2019

- Bone-anatomy, science: britannica.com, Retrieved 12 July, 2019

- Kumar, G. (15 Jul 2011). Orban's Oral Histology & Embryology (13th ed.). Elsevier India. p. 152. ISBN 9788131228197. Retrieved 1 December 2014

5

Locomotion

Locomotion is the movement of an organism from one place to another. Animal locomotion, bird flight, insect flight, aquatic locomotion, etc. fall under the study of locomotion. This chapter delves into the subject of locomotion to provide an in-depth understanding of it.

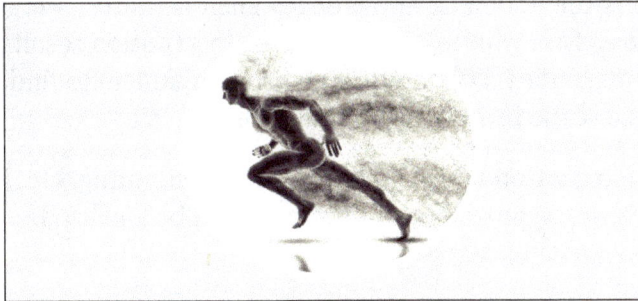

All the living organisms exhibit a special characteristic feature of moving the whole part or a part of the body from one place to another.

The act of exhibiting various motions such as running, walking, jumping, crawling, swimming, etc by the body is known as locomotion or locomotory movements.

Movement is one among the characteristic feature of all the living organisms. Locomotion helps us to move from place to other. In general, animals exhibit the locomotory movements for the sake of food and shelter.

The locomotion also helps us to run through various conditions of our environment and helps the animals to move far from their predators. The movement of the head, limbs, trunk, appendages, etc helps in changing the posture of a human body and thus maintain equilibrium condition against gravity. Consider for example- Swallowing the food implies the movement of eyeballs and external ear so that you get the information from the outside of environs.

Likewise, the movements in the heart help in the circulation of blood throughout the human body. In human beings, the locomotion and movements of the body are performed by special kind of muscles which are muscular and non-muscular in nature.

The locomotory movement in humans involves the interaction and movements of the tissues and joints such as cartilage, bone, muscles, ligaments, and tendons, etc.

Many multicellular animals consist of muscle fibres for the purpose of movements of the limbs, locomotion and also the movement of the internal organs of the body. The higher animals such as humans, there are two main systems through which the locomotion and the movements occur. The two systems are the muscular system and skeletal system. These muscles help in the movement of the appendages and the limbs.

Locomotion and Movement

Locomotion

The movement of an organism from one place to another is known as locomotion. In this process, there is the action of appendages such as limbs, wings, and flagella. In some animals, such as fish, whales, and shark, the locomotion results from a wave-like series of muscle contractions. Locomotion helps an organism to find food, avoid harsh weather conditions, escape from their predators, etc.

A few examples of locomotion are walking, running, swimming, etc. Movement, on the other hand, refers to any type of motion that need not be localized.

Movement

Movement is generally defined as a state of changing the position from rest to motion or vice-versa. Movement can be both voluntary and involuntary. Movement helps an organism to perform necessary functions, such as pumping of blood to the different parts of the body, and etc.

For example, walking is a voluntary movement, while breathing is an involuntary movement.

Difference between Locomotion and Movement

While both locomotion and movement sound similar in their meaning, there are a few interesting differences between the two terms. Let us explore these concepts better by understanding the difference between locomotion and movement:

Locomotion	Movement
Moving away from the original position of an organism is locomotion.	Movement can happen with or without moving away from an organism's original position.
It is always voluntary.	It can either be voluntary or involuntary.
Locomotion takes place at the organism level.	A movement takes place at the biological level.
Locomotion doesn't necessarily require energy	Movement requires energy.

Plants do not possess the ability to move from one place to another but various types of movement take place within plants, including phototropism, hydrotropism, geotropism, thigmotropism, etc.

Animals exhibit the most fascinating forms of movement and locomotion and this is evident from the plethora of behavioural and evolutionary traits exhibited.

For instance, one of the very first groups of organisms to take flight is the insects, which made the leap into the air roughly 412 million years ago. The very first vertebrates to take flight was the Pterosaurs, which evolved 320 million years ago. The ocean was a far more interesting place as organisms exhibited even more advanced forms of movement. Sharks, fish, whales and other aquatic species used their tails and flippers to propel themselves through the ocean, but one group of animals which includes squids and jellyfish use jet propulsion to move through the water.

ANIMAL LOCOMOTION

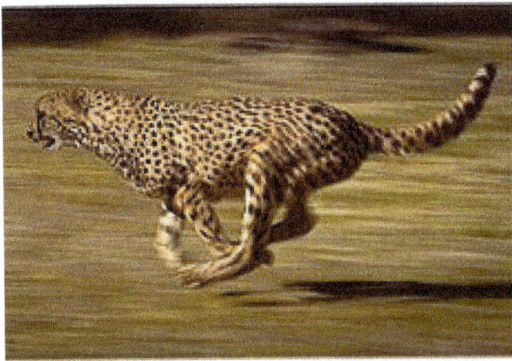

A cheetah chasing prey. In its brief hunting sprints, it is the fastest of all land animals.

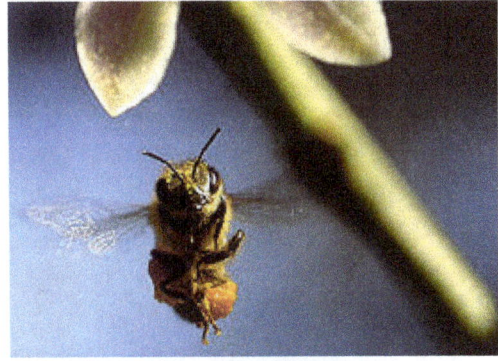

A bee in flight.

Animal locomotion, in ethology, is any of a variety of methods that animals use to move from one place to another. Some modes of locomotion are (initially) self-propelled, e.g., running, swimming, jumping, flying, hopping, soaring and gliding. There are also many animal species that depend on their environment for transportation, a type of mobility called passive locomotion, e.g., sailing (some jellyfish), kiting (spiders), rolling (some beetles and spiders) or riding other animals (phoresis).

Animals move for a variety of reasons, such as to find food, a mate, a suitable micro-habitat, or to escape predators. For many animals, the ability to move is essential for survival and, as a result, natural selection has shaped the locomotion methods and mechanisms used by moving organisms. For example, migratory animals that travel vast distances (such as the Arctic tern) typically have a locomotion mechanism that costs very little energy per unit distance, whereas non-migratory animals that must frequently move quickly to escape predators are likely to have energetically costly, but very fast, locomotion.

The anatomical structures that animals use for movement, including cilia, legs, wings, arms, fins, or tails are sometimes referred to as *locomotory organs* or *locomotory structures*.

Locomotion in Different Media

Animals move through, or on, four types of environment: aquatic (in or on water), terrestrial (on ground or other surface, including arboreal, or tree-dwelling), fossorial (underground), and aerial (in the air). Many animals—for example semi-aquatic animals, and diving birds—regularly move through more than one type of medium. In some cases, the surface they move on facilitates their method of locomotion.

Aquatic

Swimming

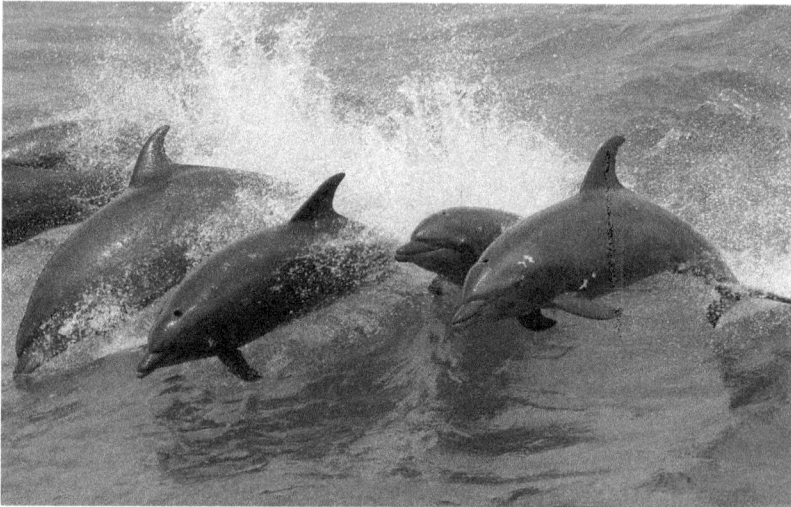

Dolphins surfing.

In water, staying afloat is possible using buoyancy. If an animal's body is less dense than water, it can stay afloat. This requires little energy to maintain a vertical position, but requires more energy for locomotion in the horizontal plane compared to less buoyant animals. The drag encountered in water is much greater than in air. Morphology is therefore important for efficient locomotion, which is in most cases essential for basic functions such as catching prey. A fusiform, torpedo-like body form is seen in many aquatic animals, though the mechanisms they use for locomotion are diverse.

The primary means by which fish generate thrust is by oscillating the body from side-to-side, the resulting wave motion ending at a large tail fin. Finer control, such as for slow movements, is often achieved with thrust from pectoral fins (or front limbs in marine mammals). Some fish, e.g. the spotted ratfish (*Hydrolagus colliei*) and batiform fish (electric rays, sawfishes, guitarfishes, skates and stingrays) use their pectoral fins as the primary means of locomotion, sometimes termed labriform swimming. Marine mammals oscillate their body in an up-and-down (dorso-ventral) direction. Other animals, e.g. penguins, diving ducks, move underwater in a manner which has been termed "aquatic flying". Some fish propel themselves without a wave motion of the body, as in the slow-moving seahorses and *Gymnotus*.

Other animals, such as cephalopods, use jet propulsion to travel fast, taking in water then squirting it back out in an explosive burst. Other swimming animals may rely predominantly on their limbs, much as humans do when swimming. Though life on land originated from the seas, terrestrial animals have returned to an aquatic lifestyle on several occasions, such as the fully aquatic cetaceans, now very distinct from their terrestrial ancestors.

Dolphins sometimes ride on the bow waves created by boats or surf on naturally breaking waves.

Benthic

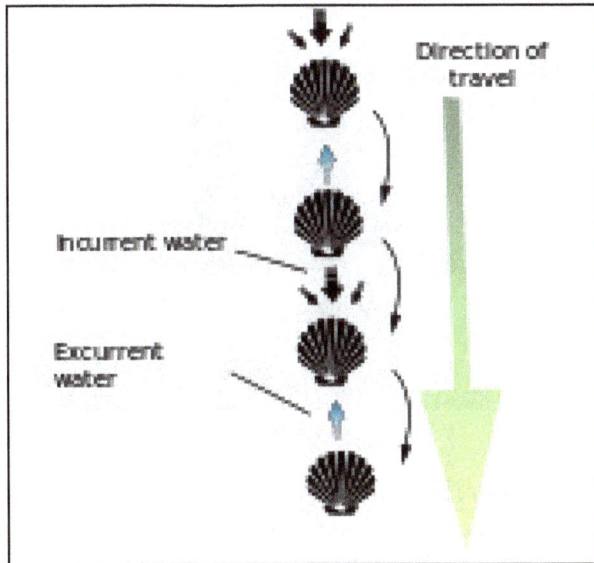

Scallop in jumping motion; these bivalves can also swim.

Benthic locomotion is movement by animals that live on, in, or near the bottom of aquatic environments. In the sea, many animals walk over the seabed. Echinoderms primarily use their tube feet to move about. The tube feet typically have a tip shaped like a suction pad that can create a vacuum through contraction of muscles. This, along with some stickiness from the secretion of mucus, provides adhesion. Waves of tube feet contractions and relaxations move along the adherent surface and the

animal moves slowly along. Some sea urchins also use their spines for benthic locomotion.

Crabs typically walk sideways (a behaviour that gives us the word *crabwise*). This is
because of the articulation of the legs, which makes a sidelong gait more efficient. However, some crabs walk forwards or backwards, including raninids, *Libinia emarginata*
and *Mictyris platycheles*. Some crabs, notably the Portunidae and Matutidae, are also
capable of swimming, the Portunidae especially so as their last pair of walking legs are
flattened into swimming paddles.

A stomatopod, *Nannosquilla decemspinosa*, can escape by rolling itself into a self-propelled wheel and somersault backwards at a speed of 72 rpm. They can travel more than
2 m using this unusual method of locomotion.

Aquatic Surface

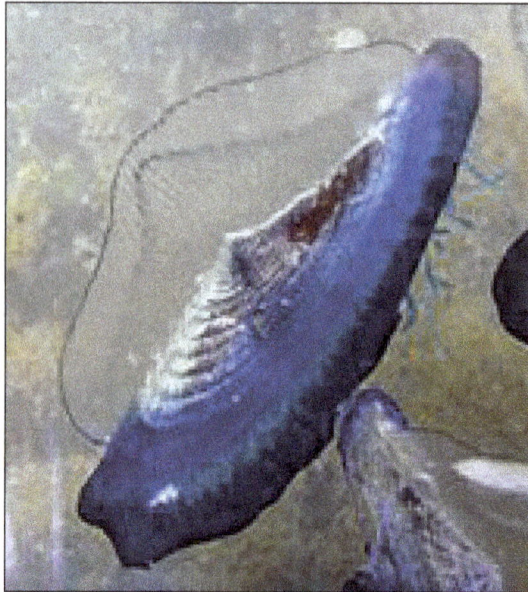

Velella moves by sailing.

Velella, the by-the-wind sailor, is a cnidarian with no means of propulsion other than
sailing. A small rigid sail projects into the air and catches the wind. *Velella* sails always
align along the direction of the wind where the sail may act as an aerofoil, so that the
animals tend to sail downwind at a small angle to the wind.

While larger animals such as ducks can move on water by floating, some small animals
move across it without breaking through the surface. This surface locomotion takes
advantage of the surface tension of water. Animals that move in such a way include the
water strider. Water striders have legs that are hydrophobic, preventing them from in-
terfering with the structure of water. Another form of locomotion (in which the surface
layer is broken) is used by the basilisk lizard.

Aerial

Active Flight

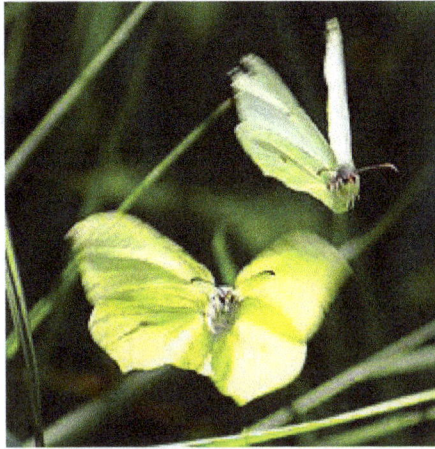

A pair of brimstone butterflies in flight. The female, above, is in fast forward
flight with a small angle of attack; the male, below, is twisting his
wings sharply upward to gain lift and fly up towards the female.

Gravity is the primary obstacle to flight. Because it is impossible for any organism to have a density as low as that of air, flying animals must generate enough lift to ascend and remain airborne. One way to achieve this is with wings, which when moved through the air generate an upward lift force on the animal's body. Flying animals must be very light to achieve flight, the largest living flying animals being birds of around 20 kilograms. Other structural adaptations of flying animals include reduced and redistributed body weight, fusiform shape and powerful flight muscles; there may also be physiological adaptations. Active flight has independently evolved at least four times, in the insects, pterosaurs, birds, and bats. Insects were the first taxon to evolve flight, approximately 400 million years ago (mya), followed by pterosaurs approximately 220 mya, birds approximately 160 mya, then bats about 60 mya.

Gliding

Rather than active flight, some (semi-) arboreal animals reduce their rate of falling by gliding. Gliding is heavier-than-air flight without the use of thrust; the term "volplaning" also refers to this mode of flight in animals. This mode of flight involves flying a greater distance horizontally than vertically and therefore can be distinguished from a simple descent like a parachute. Gliding has evolved on more occasions than active flight. There are examples of gliding animals in several major taxonomic classes such as the invertebrates (e.g., gliding ants), reptiles (e.g., banded flying snake), amphibians (e.g., flying frog), mammals (e.g., sugar glider, squirrel glider).

Some aquatic animals also regularly use gliding, for example, flying fish, octopus and squid. The flights of flying fish are typically around 50 meters (160 ft), though they can use updrafts at the leading edge of waves to cover distances of up to 400 m (1,300 ft). To glide upward out of the water, a flying fish moves its tail up to 70 times per second. Several oceanic squid, such as the Pacific flying squid, leap out of the water to escape predators, an adaptation similar to that of flying fish. Smaller squids fly in shoals, and have been observed to cover distances as long as 50 m. Small fins towards the back of the mantle help stabilize the motion of flight. They exit the water by expelling water out of their funnel, indeed some squid have been observed to continue jetting water while airborne providing thrust even after leaving the water. This may make flying squid the only animals with jet-propelled aerial locomotion. The neon flying squid has been observed to glide for distances over 30 m, at speeds of up to 11.2 m/s.

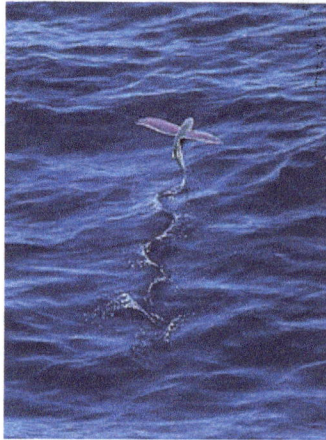

Flying fish taking off.

Soaring

Soaring birds can maintain flight without wing flapping, using rising air currents. Many gliding birds are able to "lock" their extended wings by means of a specialized tendon. Soaring birds may alternate glides with periods of soaring in rising air. Five principal types of lift are used: thermals, ridge lift, lee waves, convergences and dynamic soaring.

Examples of soaring flight by birds are the use of:

- Thermals and convergences by raptors such as vultures.

- Ridge lift by gulls near cliffs.

- Wave lift by migrating birdsDynamic effects near the surface of the sea by albatrosses.

Ballooning

Ballooning is a method of locomotion used by spiders. Certain silk-producing arthropods, mostly small or young spiders, secrete a special light-weight gossamer silk for ballooning, sometimes traveling great distances at high altitude.

Terrestrial

Forms of locomotion on land include walking, running, hopping or jumping, dragging and crawling or slithering. Here friction and buoyancy are no longer an issue, but a strong skeletal and muscular framework are required in most terrestrial animals for structural support. Each step also requires much energy to overcome inertia, and animals can store elastic potential energy in their tendons to help overcome this. Balance is also required for movement on land. Human infants learn to crawl first before they are able to stand on two feet, which requires good coordination as well as physical development. Humans are bipedal animals, standing on two feet and keeping one on the ground at all times while walking. When running, only one foot is on the ground at any one time at most, and both leave the ground briefly. At higher speeds momentum helps keep the body upright, so more energy can be used in movement.

Jumping

Jumping (saltation) can be distinguished from running, galloping, and other gaits where the entire body is temporarily airborne by the relatively long duration of the aerial phase and high angle of initial launch. Many terrestrial animals use jumping (including hopping or leaping) to escape predators or catch prey—however, relatively few animals use this as a primary mode of locomotion. Those that do include the kangaroo and other macropods, rabbit, hare, jerboa, hopping mouse, and kangaroo rat. Kangaroo rats often leap 2 m and reportedly up to 2.75 m at speeds up to almost 3 m/s (6.7 mph). They can quickly change their direction between jumps. The rapid locomotion of the banner-tailed kangaroo rat may minimize energy cost and predation risk. Its use of a "move-freeze" mode may also make it less conspicuous to nocturnal predators. Frogs are, relative to their size, the best jumpers of all vertebrates. The Australian rocket frog, *Litoria nasuta*, can leap over 2 metres (6 ft 7 in), more than fifty times its body length.

Peristalsis and Looping

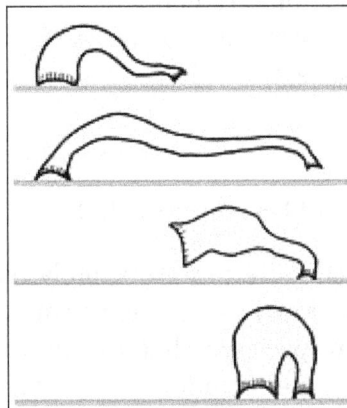

Leech moving by looping using its front and back suckers.

Other animals move in terrestrial habitats without the aid of legs. Earthworms crawl by a peristalsis, the same rhythmic contractions that propel food through the digestive tract.

Leeches and geometer moth caterpillars move by looping or inching (measuring off a length with each movement), using their paired circular and longitudinal muscles (as for peristalsis) along with the ability to attach to a surface at both anterior and posterior ends. One end is attached and the other end is projected forward peristaltically until it touches down, as far as it can reach; then the first end is released, pulled forward, and reattached; and the cycle repeats. In the case of leeches, attachment is by a sucker at each end of the body.

Sliding

Due to its low coefficient of friction, ice provides the opportunity for other modes of locomotion. Penguins either waddle on their feet or slide on their bellies across the snow, a movement called *tobogganing*, which conserves energy while moving quickly. Some pinnipeds perform a similar behaviour called *sledding*.

Climbing

Some animals are specialized for moving on non-horizontal surfaces. One common habitat for such climbing animals is in trees; for example, the gibbon is specialized for arboreal movement, travelling rapidly by brachiation.

Others living on rock faces such as in mountains move on steep or even near-vertical surfaces by careful balancing and leaping. Perhaps the most exceptional are the various types of mountain-dwelling caprids (e.g., Barbary sheep, yak, ibex, rocky mountain goat, etc.), whose adaptations can include a soft rubbery pad between their hooves for grip, hooves with sharp keratin rims for lodging in small footholds, and prominent dew claws. Another case is the snow leopard, which being a predator of such caprids also has spectacular balance and leaping abilities, such as ability to leap up to 17 m (50 ft).

Some light animals are able to climb up smooth sheer surfaces or hang upside down by adhesion using suckers. Many insects can do this, though much larger animals such as geckos can also perform similar feats.

Walking and Running

Species have different numbers of legs resulting in large differences in locomotion.

Modern birds, though classified as tetrapods, usually have only two functional legs, which some (e.g., ostrich, emu, kiwi) use as their primary, Bipedal, mode of locomotion. A few modern mammalian species are habitual bipeds, i.e., whose normal method of locomotion is two-legged. These include the macropods, kangaroo rats and mice, springhare, hopping mice, pangolins and homininan apes. Bipedalism is rarely found outside terrestrial animals—though at least two types of octopus walk bipedally on the sea floor using two of their arms, so they can use the remaining arms to camouflage themselves as a mat of algae or floating coconut.

There are no three-legged animals—though some macropods, such as kangaroos, that alternate between resting their weight on their muscular tails and their two hind legs could be looked at as an example of tripedal locomotion in animals.

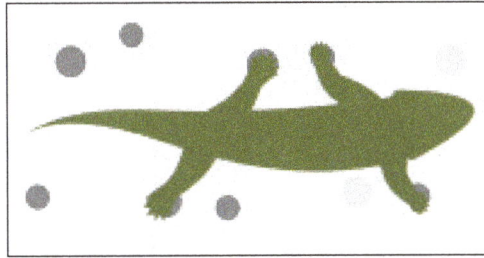

Animation of a Devonian tetrapod.

Many familiar animals are quadrupedal, walking or running on four legs. A few birds use quadrupedal movement in some circumstances. For example, the shoebill sometimes uses its wings to right itself after lunging at prey. The newly hatched hoatzin bird has claws on its thumb and first finger enabling it to dexterously climb tree branches until its wings are strong enough for sustained flight. These claws are gone by the time the bird reaches adulthood.

A relatively few animals use five limbs for locomotion. Prehensile quadrupeds may use their tail to assist in locomotion and when grazing, the kangaroos and other macropods use their tail to propel themselves forward with the four legs used to maintain balance.

Insects generally walk with six legs—though some insects such as nymphalid butterflies do not use the front legs for walking.

Arachnids have eight legs. Most arachnids lack extensor muscles in the distal joints of their appendages. Spiders and whipscorpions extend their limbs hydraulically using the pressure of their hemolymph. Solifuges and some harvestmen extend their knees by the use of highly elastic thickenings in the joint cuticle. Scorpions, pseudoscorpions and some harvestmen have evolved muscles that extend two leg joints (the femur-patella and patella-tibia joints) at once.

The scorpion *Hadrurus arizonensis* walks by using two groups of legs (left 1, right 2, Left 3, Right 4 and Right 1, Left 2, Right 3, Left 4) in a reciprocating fashion. This alternating tetrapod coordination is used over all walking speeds.

Centipedes and millipedes have many sets of legs that move in metachronal rhythm. Some echinoderms locomote using the many tube feet on the underside of their arms. Although the tube feet resemble suction cups in appearance, the gripping action is a function of adhesive chemicals rather than suction. Other chemicals and relaxation of the ampullae allow for release from the substrate. The tube feet latch on to surfaces and move in a wave, with one arm section attaching to the surface as another releases. Some multi-armed, fast-moving starfish such as the sunflower seastar (*Pycnopodia helianthoides*) pull themselves along with some of their arms while letting others trail behind. Other starfish turn up the tips of their arms while moving, which exposes the sensory tube feet and eyespot to external stimuli. Most starfish cannot move quickly, a typical speed being that of the leather star (*Dermasterias imbricata*), which can manage just 15 cm (6 in) in a minute. Some burrowing species from the genera *Astropecten* and *Luidia* have points rather than suckers on their long tube feet and are capable of much more rapid motion, "gliding" across the ocean floor. The sand star (*Luidia foliolata*) can travel at a speed of 2.8 m (9 ft 2 in) per minute. Sunflower starfish are quick, efficient hunters, moving at a speed of 1 m/min (3.3 ft/min) using 15,000 tube feet.

Many animals temporarily change the number of legs they use for locomotion in different circumstances. For example, many quadrupedal animals switch to bipedalism to reach low-level browse on trees. The genus of *Basiliscus* are arboreal lizards that usually use quadrupedalism in the trees. When frightened, they can drop to water below and run across the surface on their hind limbs at about 1.5 m/s for a distance of approximately 4.5 m (15 ft) before they sink to all fours and swim. They can also sustain themselves on all fours while "water-walking" to increase the distance travelled above the surface by about 1.3 m. When cockroaches run rapidly, they rear up on their two hind legs like bipedal humans; this allows them to run at speeds up to 50 body lengths per second, equivalent to a "couple hundred miles per hour, if you scale up to the size of humans." When grazing, kangaroos use a form of pentapedalism (four legs plus the tail) but switch to hopping (bipedalism) when they wish to move at a greater speed.

Powered Cartwheeling

The Moroccan flic-flac spider (Cebrennus rechenbergi) uses a series of rapid, acrobatic flic-flac movements of its legs similar to those used by gymnasts, to actively propel itself off the ground, allowing it to move both down and uphill, even at a 40 percent incline. This behaviour is different than other huntsman spiders, such as Carparachne aureoflava from the Namib Desert, which uses passive cartwheeling as a form of locomotion. The flic-flac spider can reach speeds of up to 2 m/s using forward or back flips to evade threats.

Subterranean

Some animals move through solids such as soil by burrowing using peristalsis, as in earthworms, or other methods. In loose solids such as sand some animals, such as the golden mole, marsupial mole, and the pink fairy armadillo, are able to move more rapidly, "swimming" through the loose substrate. Burrowing animals include moles, ground squirrels, naked mole-rats, tilefish, and mole crickets.

Energetics

Animal locomotion requires energy to overcome various forces including friction, drag, inertia and gravity, although the influence of these depends on the circumstances. In terrestrial environments, gravity must be overcome whereas the drag of air has little influence. In aqueous environments, friction (or drag) becomes the major energetic challenge with gravity being less of an influence. Remaining in the aqueous environment, animals with natural buoyancy expend little energy to maintain a vertical position in a water column. Others naturally sink, and must spend energy to remain afloat. Drag is also an energetic influence in flight, and the aerodynamically efficient body shapes of flying birds indicate how they have evolved to cope with this. Limbless organisms moving on land must energetically overcome surface friction, however, they do not usually need to expend significant energy to counteract gravity.

Newton's third law of motion is widely used in the study of animal locomotion: if at rest, to move forwards an animal must push something backwards. Terrestrial animals must push the solid ground, swimming and flying animals must push against a fluid (either water or air). The effect of forces during locomotion on the design of the skeletal system is also important, as is the interaction between locomotion and muscle physiology, in determining how the structures and effectors of locomotion enable or limit animal movement. The energetics of locomotion involves the energy expenditure by animals in moving. Energy consumed in locomotion is not available for other efforts, so animals typically have evolved to use the minimum energy possible during movement. However, in the case of certain behaviors, such as locomotion to escape a predator, performance (such as speed or maneuverability) is more crucial, and such movements may be energetically expensive. Furthermore, animals may use energetically expensive methods of locomotion when environmental conditions (such as being within a burrow) preclude other modes.

The most common metric of energy use during locomotion is the net (also termed "incremental") cost of transport, defined as the amount of energy (e.g., Joules) needed above baseline metabolic rate to move a given distance. For aerobic locomotion, most animals have a nearly constant cost of transport—moving a given distance requires the same caloric expenditure, regardless of speed. This constancy is usually accomplished by changes in gait. The net cost of transport of swimming is lowest, followed by flight, with terrestrial limbed locomotion being the most expensive per unit distance. However, because of the speeds involved, flight requires the most energy per unit time. This does not mean that an animal that normally moves by running would be a more efficient swimmer; however, these comparisons assume an animal is specialized for that form of motion. Another consideration here is body mass—heavier animals, though using more total energy, require less energy *per unit mass* to move. Physiologists generally measure energy use by the amount of oxygen consumed, or the amount of carbon dioxide produced, in an animal's respiration. In terrestrial animals, the cost of transport is typically measured while they walk or run on a motorized treadmill, either wearing a mask to capture gas exchange or with the entire treadmill enclosed in a metabolic chamber. For small rodents, such as deer mice, the cost of transport has also been measured during voluntary wheel running.

Energetics is important for explaining the evolution of foraging economic decisions in organisms; for example, a study of the African honey bee, *A. m. scutellata*, has shown that honey bees may trade the high sucrose content of viscous nectar off for the energetic benefits of warmer, less concentrated nectar, which also reduces their consumption and flight time.

Passive Locomotion

Passive locomotion in animals is a type of mobility in which the animal depends on their environment for transportation.

Hydrozoans

The Portuguese man o' war (Physalia physalis) lives at the surface of the ocean. The gas-filled bladder, or pneumatophore (sometimes called a "sail"), remains at the surface, while the remainder is submerged. Because the Portuguese man o' war has no means of propulsion, it is moved by a combination of winds, currents, and tides. The sail is equipped with a siphon. In the event of a surface attack, the sail can be deflated, allowing the organism to briefly submerge.

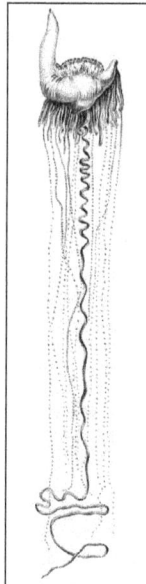

Physalia physalis.

Arachnids

The wheel spider (*Carparachne aureoflava*) is a huntsman spider approximately 20 mm in size and native to the Namib Desert of Southern Africa. The spider escapes parasitic pompilid wasps by flipping onto its side and cartwheeling down sand dunes at speeds of up to 44 turns per second. If the spider is on a sloped dune, its rolling speed may be 1 metre per second.

A spider (usually limited to individuals of a small species), or spiderling after hatching, climbs as high as it can, stands on raised legs with its abdomen pointed upwards ("tip-toeing"), and then releases several silk threads from its spinnerets into the air. These form a triangle-shaped parachute that carries the spider on updrafts of winds, where even the slightest breeze transports it. The Earth's static electric field may also provide lift in windless conditions.

Insects

The larva of *Cicindela dorsalis*, the eastern beach tiger beetle, is notable for its ability to leap into the air, loop its body into a rotating wheel and roll along the sand at a high speed using wind to propel itself. If the wind is strong enough, the larva can cover up to 60 metres (200 ft) in this manner. This remarkable ability may have evolved to help the larva escape predators such as the thynnid wasp *Methocha*.

Members of the largest subfamily of cuckoo wasps, Chrysidinae, are generally klepto-parasites, laying their eggs in host nests, where their larvae consume the host egg or larva while it is still young. Chrysidines are distinguished from the members of other subfamilies in that most have flattened or concave lower abdomens and can curl into a defensive ball when attacked by a potential host, a process known as conglobation. Protected by hard chitin in this position, they are expelled from the nest without injury and can search for a less hostile host.

Fleas can jump vertically up to 18 cm and horizontally up to 33 cm; however, although this form of locomotion is initiated by the flea, it has little control of the jump—they always jump in the same direction, with very little variation in the trajectory between individual jumps.

Crustaceans

Although stomatopods typically display the standard locomotion types as seen in true shrimp and lobsters, one species, *Nannosquilla decemspinosa*, has been observed flipping itself into a crude wheel. The species lives in shallow, sandy areas. At low tides, *N. decemspinosa* is often stranded by its short rear legs, which are sufficient for locomotion when the body is supported by water, but not on dry land. The mantis shrimp then performs a forward flip in an attempt to roll towards the next tide pool. *N. decemspinosa* has been observed to roll repeatedly for 2 m (6.6 ft), but they typically travel less than 1 m (3.3 ft). Again, the animal initiates the movement but has little control during its locomotion.

Animal Transport

Some animals change location because they are attached to, or reside on, another animal or moving structure. This is arguably more accurately termed "animal transport".

Remoras

Remoras are a family (*Echeneidae*) of ray-finned fish. They grow to 30–90 cm (0.98–2.95 ft) long, and their distinctive first dorsal fins take the form of a modified oval, sucker-like organ with slat-like structures that open and close to create suction and take a firm hold against the skin of larger marine animals. By sliding backward, the remora can increase the suction, or it can release itself by swimming forward. Remoras sometimes attach to small boats. They swim well on their own, with a sinuous, or curved, motion. When the remora reaches about 3 cm (1.2 in), the disc is fully formed and the remora can then attach to other animals. The remora's lower jaw projects beyond the upper, and the animal lacks a swim bladder. Some remoras associate primarily with specific host species. They are commonly found attached to sharks, manta rays, whales, turtles, and dugongs. Smaller remoras also fasten onto fish such as tuna and swordfish, and some small remoras travel in the mouths or gills of large manta rays, ocean sunfish, swordfish, and sailfish. The remora benefits by using the host as transport and protection, and also feeds on materials dropped by the host.

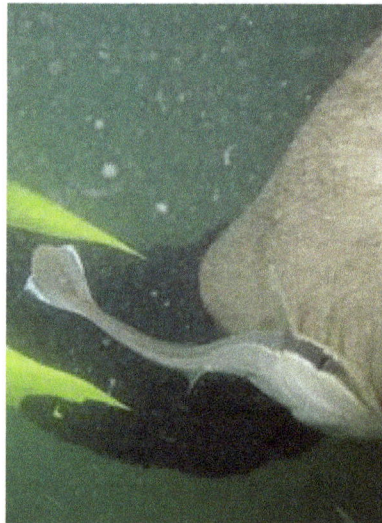

Some remoras, such as this *Echeneis naucrates*, may attach themselves to scuba divers.

Angler Fish

In some species of anglerfish, when a male finds a female, he bites into her skin, and releases an enzyme that digests the skin of his mouth and her body, fusing the pair down to the blood-vessel level. The male becomes dependent on the female host for survival by receiving nutrients via their shared circulatory system, and provides sperm to the female in return. After fusing, males increase in volume and become much larger relative to free-living males of the species. They live and remain reproductively functional as long as the female lives, and can take part in multiple spawnings. This extreme sexual dimorphism ensures, when the female is ready to spawn, she has a mate immediately available. Multiple males can be incorporated into a single individual female with up to eight males in some species, though some taxa appear to have a one male per female rule.

Parasites

Many parasites are transported by their hosts. For example, endoparasites such as tapeworms live in the alimentary tracts of other animals, and depend on the host's ability to move to distribute their eggs. Ectoparasites such as fleas can move around on the body of their host, but are transported much longer distances by the host's locomotion. Some ectoparasites such as lice can opportunistically hitch a ride on a fly (phoresis) and attempt to find a new host.

Changes between Media

Some animals locomote between different media, e.g., from aquatic to aerial. This often requires different modes of locomotion in the different media and may require a distinct transitional locomotor behaviour.

There are a large number of semi-aquatic animals (animals that spend part of their life cycle in water, or generally have part of their anatomy underwater). These represent the major taxons of mammals (e.g., beaver, otter, polar bear), birds (e.g., penguins, ducks), reptiles (e.g., anaconda, bog turtle, marine iguana) and amphibians (e.g., salamanders, frogs, newts).

Fish

Some fish use multiple modes of locomotion. Walking fish may swim freely or at other times "walk" along the ocean or river floor, but not on land (e.g., the flying gurnard—which does not actually fly—and batfishes of the family Ogcocephalidae). Amphibious fish, are fish that are able to leave water for extended periods of time. These fish use a range of terrestrial locomotory modes, such as lateral undulation, tripod-like walking (using paired fins and tail), and jumping. Many of these locomotory modes incorporate multiple combinations of pectoral, pelvic and tail fin movement. Examples include eels, mudskippers and the walking catfish. Flying fish can make powerful, self-propelled leaps out of water into air, where their long, wing-like fins enable gliding flight for considerable distances above the water's surface. This uncommon ability is a natural defence mechanism to evade predators. The flights of flying fish are typically around 50 m, though they can use updrafts at the leading edge of waves to cover distances of up to 400 m (1,300 ft). They can travel at speeds of more than 70 km/h (43 mph). Maximum altitude is 6 m (20 ft) above the surface of the sea. Some accounts have them landing on ships' decks.

Marine Mammals

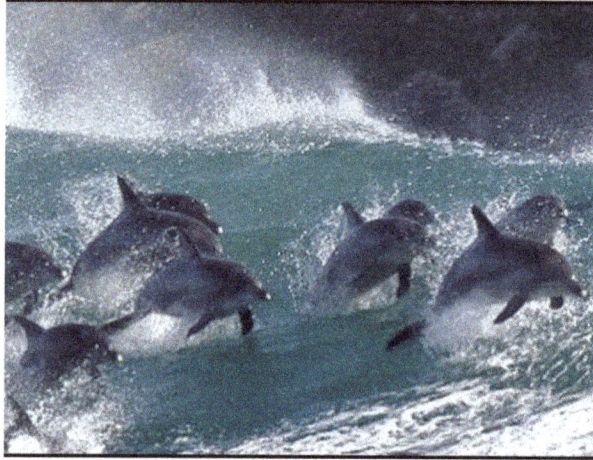
Pacific white-sided dolphins porpoising.

When swimming, several marine mammals such as dolphins, porpoises and pinnipeds, frequently leap above the water surface whilst maintaining horizontal locomotion. This is done for various reasons. When travelling, jumping can save dolphins and porpoises energy as there is less friction while in the air. This type of travel is known as "porpoising". Other reasons for dolphins and porpoises performing porpoising include orientation, social displays, fighting, non-verbal communication, entertainment and attempting to dislodge parasites. In pinnipeds, two types of porpoising have been identified. "High porpoising" is most often near (within 100 m) the shore and is often followed by minor course changes; this may help seals get their bearings on beaching or rafting sites. "Low porpoising" is typically observed relatively far (more than 100 m) from shore and often aborted in favour of anti-predator movements; this may be a way for seals to maximize sub-surface vigilance and thereby reduce their vulnerability to sharks.

Some whales raise their (entire) body vertically out of the water in a behaviour known as "breaching".

Birds

Some semi-aquatic birds use terrestrial locomotion, surface swimming, underwater swimming and flying (e.g., ducks, swans). Diving birds also use diving locomotion (e.g., dippers, auks). Some birds (e.g., ratites) have lost the primary locomotion of flight. The largest of these, ostriches, when being pursued by a predator, have been known to reach speeds over 70 km/h (43 mph), and can maintain a steady speed of 50 km/h (31 mph), which makes the ostrich the world's fastest two-legged animal: Ostriches can also locomote by swimming. Penguins either waddle on their feet or slide on their bellies across the snow, a movement called *tobogganing*, which conserves energy while moving quickly. They also jump with both feet together if they want to move more quickly or cross steep or rocky terrain. To get onto land, penguins sometimes propel themselves upwards at a great speed to leap out the water.

Changes during the Life-cycle

An animal's mode of locomotion may change considerably during its life-cycle. Barnacles are exclusively marine and tend to live in shallow and tidal waters. They have two nektonic (active swimming) larval stages, but as adults, they are sessile (non-motile) suspension feeders. Frequently, adults are found attached to moving objects such as whales and ships, and are thereby transported (passive locomotion) around the oceans.

Function

Animals locomote for a variety of reasons, such as to find food, a mate, a suitable microhabitat, or to escape predators.

Food Procurement

Animals use locomotion in a wide variety of ways to procure food. Terrestrial methods include ambush predation, social predation and grazing. Aquatic methods include filterfeeding, grazing, ram feeding, suction feeding, protrusion and pivot feeding. Other methods include parasitism and parasitoidism.

Methods of Study

A variety of methods and equipment are used to study animal locomotion:

- Treadmills are used to allow animals to walk or run while remaining stationary with respect to external observers. This technique facilitates filming or recordings of physiological information from the animal (e.g., during studies of energetics). Motorized treadmills are also used to measure the endurance capacity (stamina) of animals.

- Racetracks lined with photocells or filmed while animals run along them are used to measure acceleration and maximal sprint speed.

- Kinematics is the study of the motion of an entire animal or parts of its body. It is typically accomplished by placing visual markers at particular anatomical locations on the animal and then recording video of its movement. The video is often captured from multiple angles, with frame rates exceeding 2000 frames per second when capturing high speed movement. The location of each marker is determined for each video frame, and data from multiple views is integrated to give positions of each point through time. Computers are sometimes used to track the markers, although this task must often be performed manually. The kinematic data can be used to determine fundamental motion attributes such as velocity, acceleration, joint angles, and the sequencing and timing of kinematic events. These fundamental attributes can be used to quantify various higher level attributes, such as the physical abilities of the animal (e.g., its maximum running speed, how steep a slope it can climb), neural control of locomotion, gait, and responses to environmental variation. These, in turn, can aid in formulation of hypotheses about the animal or locomotion in general.

- Force plates are platforms, usually part of a trackway, that can be used to measure the magnitude and direction of forces of an animal's step. When used with kinematics and a sufficiently detailed model of anatomy, inverse dynamics solutions can determine the forces not just at the contact with the ground, but at each joint in the limb.

- Electromyography (EMG) is a method of detecting the electrical activity that occurs when muscles are activated, thus determining which muscles an animal uses for a given movement. This can be accomplished either by surface electrodes (usually in large animals) or implanted electrodes (often wires thinner than a human hair). Furthermore, the intensity of electrical activity can correlate to the level of muscle activity, with greater activity implying (though not definitively showing) greater force.

- Sonomicrometry employs a pair of piezoelectric crystals implanted in a muscle or tendon to continuously measure the length of a muscle or tendon. This is useful because surface kinematics may be inaccurate due to skin movement. Similarly, if an elastic tendon is in series with the muscle, the muscle length may not be accurately reflected by the joint angle.

- Tendon force buckles measure the force produced by a single muscle by measuring the strain of a tendon. After the experiment, the tendon's elastic modulus is determined and used to compute the exact force produced by the muscle. However, this can only be used on muscles with long tendons.

- Particle image velocimetry is used in aquatic and aerial systems to measure the flow of fluid around and past a moving aquatic organism, allowing fluid dynamics calculations to determine pressure gradients, speeds, etc.

- Fluoroscopy allows real-time X-ray video, for precise kinematics of moving bones. Markers opaque to X-rays can allow simultaneous tracking of muscle length.

These methods can be combined. For example, studies frequently combine EMG and kinematics to determine *motor pattern*, the series of electrical and kinematic events that produce a given movement.

BIRD FLIGHT

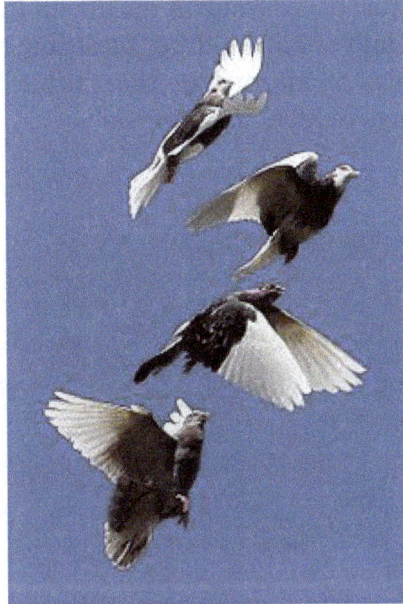

A flock of domestic pigeons each in a different phase of its flap.

Bird flight is the primary mode of locomotion used by most bird species in which birds take off and fly. Flight assists birds with feeding, breeding, avoiding predators, and migrating.

Bird flight is one of the most complex forms of locomotion in the animal kingdom. Each facet of this type of motion, including hovering, taking off, and landing, involves many complex movements. As different bird species adapted over millions of years through evolution for specific environments, prey, predators, and other needs, they developed specializations in their wings, and acquired different forms of flight.

Various theories exist about how bird flight evolved, including flight from falling or gliding (the *trees down* hypothesis), from running or leaping (the *ground up* hypothesis), from *wing-assisted incline running* or from *proavis* (pouncing) behavior.

Basic Mechanics of Bird Flight

Lift and Drag

The fundamentals of bird flight are similar to those of aircraft, in which the aerodynamic forces sustaining flight are lift and drag. Lift force is produced by the action of air flow on the wing, which is an airfoil. The airfoil is shaped such that the air provides a net upward force on the wing, while the movement of air is directed downward. Additional net lift may come from airflow around the bird's body in some species, especially during intermittent flight while the wings are folded or semi-folded.

Aerodynamic drag is the force opposite to the direction of motion, and hence the source of energy loss in flight. The drag force can be separated into two portions, *lift-induced drag*, which is the inherent cost of the wing producing lift (this energy ends up primarily in the wingtip vortices), and *parasitic drag*, including skin friction drag from the friction of air and body surfaces and form drag from the bird's frontal area. The streamlining of bird's body and wings reduces these forces.

Wings

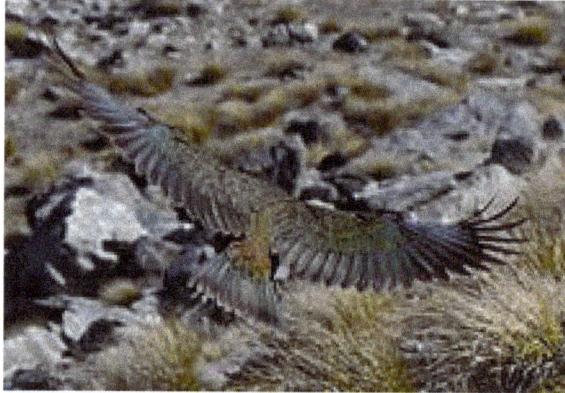
A kea in flight.

The bird's forelimbs (the wings) are the key to flight. Each wing has a central vane to hit the wind, composed of three limb bones, the humerus, ulna and radius. The hand, or manus, which ancestrally was composed of five digits, is reduced to three digits, which serves as an anchor for the primaries, one of two groups of flight feathers responsible for the wing's airfoil shape. The other set of flight feathers, behind the carpal joint on the ulna, are called the secondaries. The remaining feathers on the wing are known as coverts, of which there are three sets. The wing sometimes has vestigial claws. In most species, these are lost by the time the bird is adult (such as the highly visible ones used for active climbing by hoatzin chicks), but claws are retained into adulthood by the secretarybird, screamers, finfoots, ostriches, several swifts and numerous others, as a local trait, in a few specimens.

Albatrosses have locking mechanisms in the wing joints that reduce the strain on the muscles during soaring flight.

Even within a species wing morphology may differ. For example, adult European Turtle Doves have been found to have longer but more rounded wings than juveniles – suggesting that juvenile wing morphology facilitates their first migrations, while selection for flight maneuverability is more important after the juveniles' first molt.

Female birds exposed to predators during ovulation produce chicks that grow their wings faster than chicks produced by predator-free females. Their wings are also longer. Both adaptations may make them better at avoiding avian predators.

Wing Shape

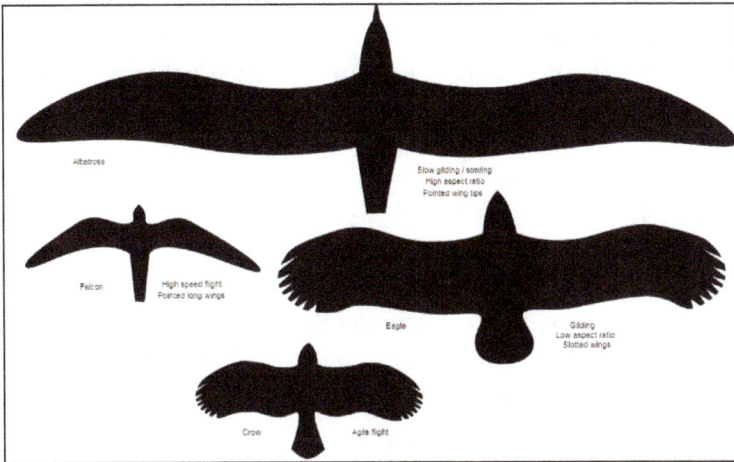

Wing shapes.

The shape of the wing is important in determining the flight capabilities of a bird. Different shapes correspond to different trade-offs between advantages such as speed, low energy use, and maneuverability. Two important parameters are the aspect ratio and wing loading. Aspect ratio is the ratio of wingspan to the mean of its chord (or the square of the wingspan divided by wing area). Wing loading is the ratio of weight to wing area.

Most kinds of bird wing can be grouped into four types, with some falling between two of these types. These types of wings are elliptical wings, high speed wings, high aspect ratio wings and soaring wings with slots.

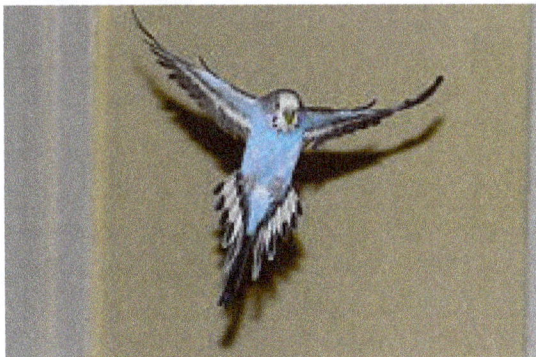

The budgerigar's wings, as seen on this pet female, allow it excellent manoeuvrability.

Elliptical Wings

Technically, elliptical wings are those having elliptical (that is quarter ellipses) meeting conformally at the tips. The early model Supermarine Spitfire is an example. Some birds have vaguely elliptical wings, including the albatross wing of high aspect ratio. Although the term is convenient, it might be more precise to refer to curving taper with fairly small radius at the tips. Many small birds have having a low aspect ratio with elliptical character (when spread), allowing for tight maneuvering in confined spaces such as might be found in dense vegetation. As such they are common in forest raptors (such as *Accipiter* hawks), and many passerines, particularly non-migratory ones (migratory species have longer wings). They are also common in species that use a rapid take off to evade predators, such as pheasants and partridges.

High Speed Wings

High speed wings are short, pointed wings that when combined with a heavy wing loading and rapid wingbeats provide an energetically expensive, but high speed. This type of flight is used by the bird with the fastest wing speed, the peregrine falcon, as well as by most of the ducks. The same wing shape is used by the auks for a different purpose; auks use their wings to "fly" underwater.

The peregrine falcon has the highest recorded dive speed of 242 mph (389 km/h). The fastest straight, powered flight is the spine-tailed swift at 105 mph (170 km/h).

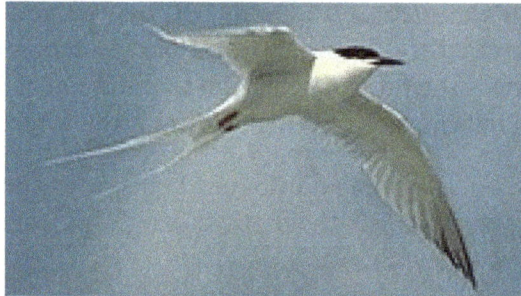

A roseate tern uses its low wing loading and
high aspect ratio to achieve low speed flight.

High Aspect Ratio Wings

High aspect ratio wings, which usually have low wing loading and are far longer than they are wide, are used for slower flight. This may take the form of almost hovering (as used by kestrels, terns and nightjars) or in soaring and gliding flight, particularly the dynamic soaring used by seabirds, which takes advantage of wind speed variation at different altitudes (wind shear) above ocean waves to provide lift. Low speed flight is also important for birds that plunge-dive for fish.

Soaring Wings with Deep Slots

These wings are favored by larger species of inland birds, such as eagles, vultures, pelicans, and storks. The slots at the end of the wings, between the primaries, reduce the induced drag and wingtip vortices by "capturing" the energy in air flowing from the lower to upper wing surface at the tips, whilst the shorter size of the wings aids in take-off (high aspect ratio wings require a long taxi to get airborne).

Flight

Birds use three types of flight. They are distinguished by wing motion.

Gliding Flight

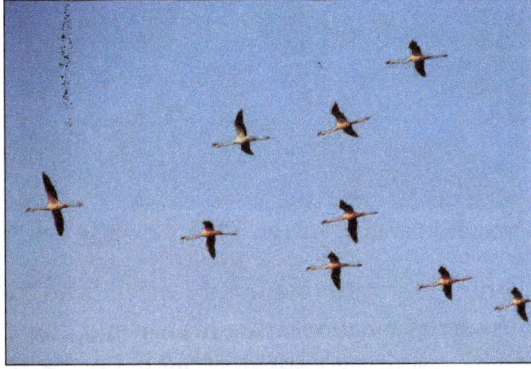

Lesser flamingos flying in formation.

When in gliding flight, the upward aerodynamic force is equal to the weight. In gliding flight, no propulsion is used; the energy to counteract the energy loss due to aerodynamic drag is either taken from the potential energy of the bird, resulting in a descending flight, or is replaced by rising air currents ("thermals"), referred to as soaring flight. For specialist soaring birds (obligate soarers), the decision to engage in flight are strongly related to atmospheric conditions that allow individuals to maximise flight-efficiency and minimise energetic costs.

Flapping Flight

When a bird flaps, as opposed to gliding, its wings continue to develop lift as before, but the lift is rotated forward to provide thrust, which counteracts drag and increases its speed, which has the effect of also increasing lift to counteract its weight, allowing it to maintain height or to climb. Flapping involves two stages: the down-stroke, which provides the majority of the thrust, and the up-stroke, which can also (depending on the bird's wings) provide some thrust. At each up-stroke the wing is slightly folded inwards to reduce the energetic cost of flapping-wing flight. Birds change the angle of attack continuously within a flap, as well as with speed.

Bounding Flight

Small birds often fly long distances using a technique in which short bursts of flapping are alternated with intervals in which the wings are folded against the body. This is a flight pattern known as "bounding" or "flap-bounding" flight. When the bird's wings are folded, its trajectory is primarily ballistic, with a small amount of body lift. The flight pattern is believed to decrease the energy required by reducing the aerodynamic drag during the ballistic part of the trajectory, and to increase the efficiency of muscle use.

Hovering

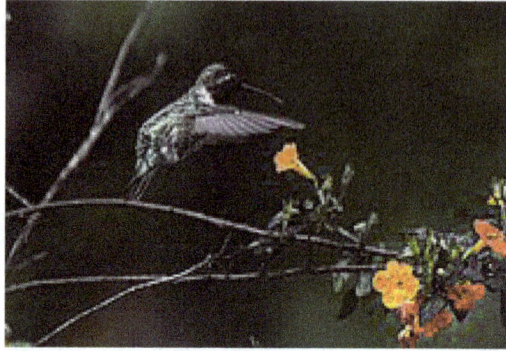

The ruby-throated hummingbird can beat its wings 52 times a second.

Several bird species use hovering, with one family specialized for hovering – the hummingbirds. True hovering occurs by generating lift through flapping alone, rather than by passage through the air, requiring considerable energy expenditure. This usually confines the ability to smaller birds, but some larger birds, such as a kite or osprey can hover for a short period of time. Although not a true hover, some birds remain in a fixed position relative to the ground or water by flying into a headwind. Hummingbirds, kestrels, terns and hawks use this wind hovering.

Most birds that hover have high aspect ratio wings that are suited to low speed flying. Hummingbirds are a unique exception – the most accomplished hoverers of all birds. Hummingbird flight is different from other bird flight in that the wing is extended throughout the whole stroke, which is a symmetrical figure of eight, with the wing producing lift on both the up- and down-stroke. Hummingbirds beat their wings at some 43 times per second, while others may be as high as 80 times per second.

Take-off and Landing

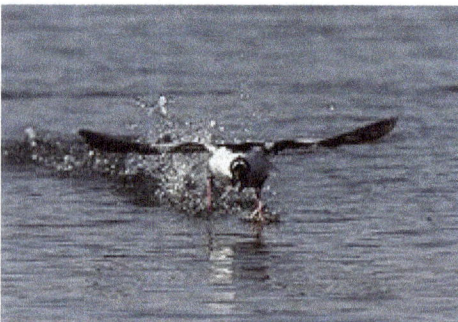

A male bufflehead runs atop the water while taking off.

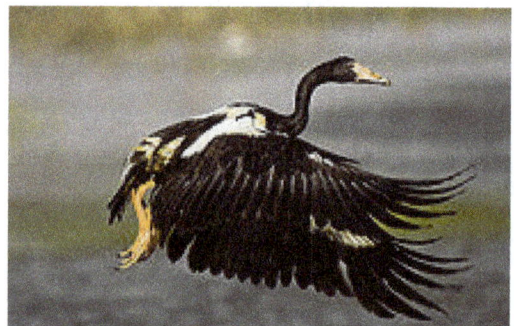

A magpie-goose taking off.

Take-off is one of the most energetically demanding aspects of flight, as the bird must generate enough airflow across the wing to create lift. Small birds do this with a simple upward jump. That doesn't work for larger birds, which must take a run up to generate sufficient airflow. Large birds take off by facing into the wind, or, if they can, by perching on a branch or cliff so they can just drop off into the air.

Landing is also a problem for large birds with high wing loads. This problem is dealt with in some species by aiming for a point below the intended landing area (such as a nest on a cliff) then pulling up beforehand. If timed correctly, the airspeed once the target is reached is virtually nil. Landing on water is simpler, and the larger waterfowl species prefer to do so whenever possible, landing into wind and using their feet as skids. To lose height rapidly prior to landing, some large birds such as geese indulge in a rapid alternating series of sideslips or even briefly turning upside down in a maneuver termed as whiffling.

Coordinated Formation Flight

A wide variety of birds fly together in a symmetric V-shaped or a J-shaped coordinated formation, also referred to as an "echelon", especially during long distance flight or migration. It is often assumed that birds resort to this pattern of formation flying in order to save energy and improve the aerodynamic efficiency. The birds flying at the tips and at the front would interchange positions in a timely cyclical fashion to spread flight fatigue equally among the flock members.

The wingtips of the leading bird in an echelon create a pair of opposite rotating line vortices. The vortices trailing a bird have an underwash part behind the bird, and at the same time they have an upwash on the outside, that hypothetically could aid the flight of a trailing bird. In a 1970 study the authors claimed that each bird in a V formation of 25 members can achieve a reduction of induced drag and as a result increase their range by 71%.

Studies of waldrapp ibis show that birds spatially coordinate the phase of wing flapping and show wingtip path coherence when flying in V positions, thus enabling them to maximally utilise the available energy of upwash over the entire flap cycle. In contrast, birds flying in a stream immediately behind another do not have wingtip coherence in their flight pattern and their flapping is out of phase, as compared to birds flying in V patterns, so as to avoid the detrimental effects of the downwash due to the leading bird's flight.

Adaptations for Flight

The most obvious adaptation to flight is the wing, but because flight is so energetically demanding birds have evolved several other adaptations to improve efficiency when flying. Birds' bodies are streamlined to help overcome air-resistance. Also, the bird skeleton is hollow to reduce weight, and many unnecessary bones have been lost (such as the bony tail of the early bird *Archaeopteryx*), along with the toothed jaw of early birds, which has been replaced with a lightweight beak. The skeleton's breastbone has also adapted into a large keel, suitable for the attachment of large, powerful flight muscles. The vanes of each feather have hooklets called barbules that zip the vanes of individual feathers together, giving the feathers the strength needed to hold the airfoil (these are often lost in flightless birds). The barbules maintain the shape and function of the feather. Each feather has a major (greater) side and a minor (lesser) side, meaning that the shaft or rachis does not run down the center of the feather. Rather it runs longitudinally of center with the lesser or minor side to the front and the greater or major side to the rear of the feather. This feather anatomy, during flight and flapping of the wings, causes a rotation of the feather in its follicle. The rotation occurs in the up motion of the wing. The greater side points down, letting air slip through the wing. This essentially breaks the integrity of the wing, allowing for a much easier movement in the up direction. The integrity of the wing is reestablished in the down movement, which allows for part of the lift inherent in bird wings. This function is most important in taking off or achieving lift at very low or slow speeds where the bird is reaching up and grabbing air and pulling itself up. At high speeds the air foil function of the wing provides most of the lift needed to stay in flight.

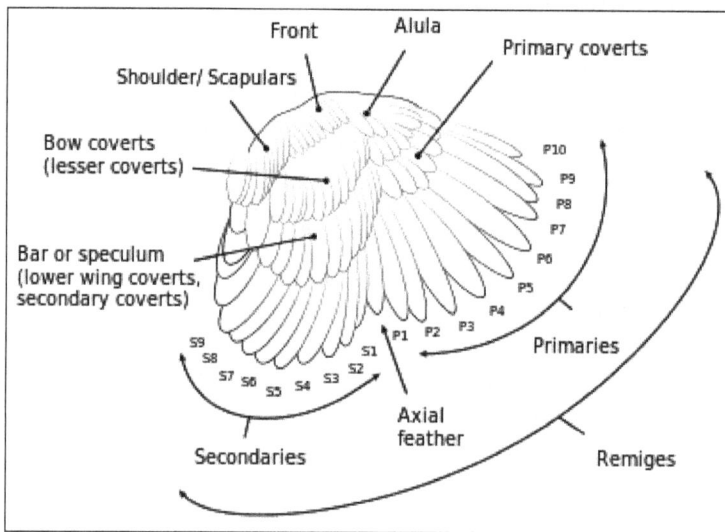

Diagram of the wing of a chicken, top view.

The large amounts of energy required for flight have led to the evolution of a unidirectional pulmonary system to provide the large quantities of oxygen required for their high respiratory rates. This high metabolic rate produces large quantities of radicals in the cells that can damage DNA and lead to tumours. Birds, however, do not suffer from an otherwise expected shortened lifespan as their cells have evolved a more efficient antioxidant system than those found in other animals.

INSECT FLIGHT

Insects are the only group of invertebrates that have evolved wings and flight. Two insect groups, the dragonflies and the mayflies, have flight muscles attached directly to the wings. Other insects have the flight muscles attached to the thorax, making it oscillate, sometimes at a faster rate than the arrival rate of nerve impulses, and indirectly causing the wings to beat.

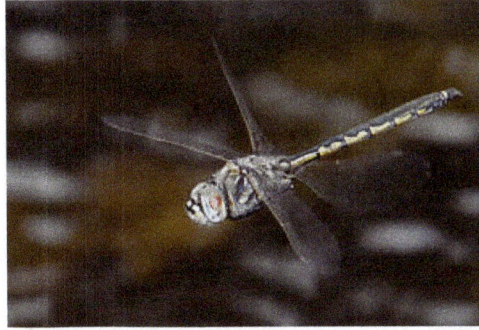

A tau emerald (*Hemicordulia tau*) dragonfly has
flight muscles attached directly to its wings.

Some very small insects make use not of steady-state aerodynamics but of the Weis-Fogh clap and fling mechanism, generating large lift forces at the expense of wear and tear on the wings. Many insects can hover, maintaining height and controlling their position. Some insects such as moths have the forewings coupled to the hindwings so these can work in unison.

Insects first flew in the Carboniferous, some 350 million years ago. Wings may have evolved from appendages on the sides of existing limbs, which already had nerves, joints, and muscles used for other purposes. These may initially have been used for sailing on water, or to slow the rate of descent when gliding.

Mechanisms

Direct Flight

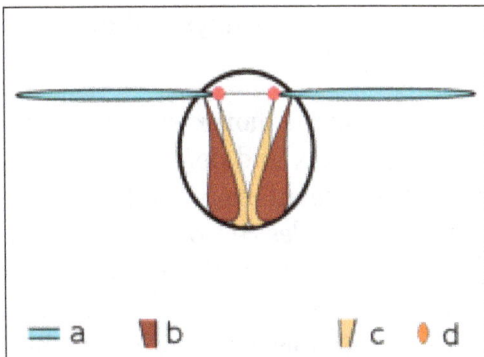

Direct flight: muscles attached to wings.
Large insects only.

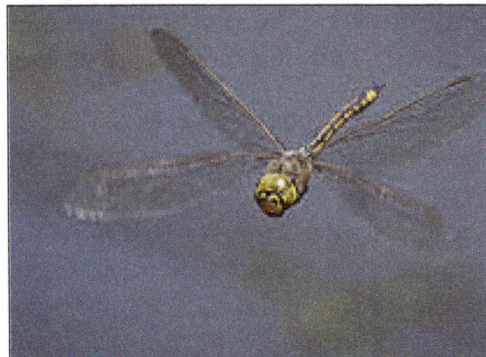

The Odonata (dragonflies and damselflies)
have direct flight musculature, as do mayflies.

Unlike other insects, the wing muscles of the Ephemeroptera (mayflies) and Odonata (dragonflies and damselflies) insert directly at the wing bases, which are hinged so that a small movement of the wing base downward, lifts the wing itself upward, very much like rowing through the air. Dragonflies and damselflies have fore and hind wings similar in shape and size. Each operates independently, which gives a degree of fine control and mobility in terms of the abruptness with which they can change direction and speed, not seen in other flying insects. This is not surprising, given that odonates are all aerial predators, and they have always hunted other airborne insects.

Indirect Flight

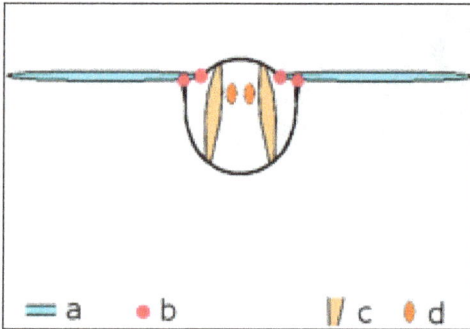

Indirect flight: muscles make thorax oscillate in most insects.

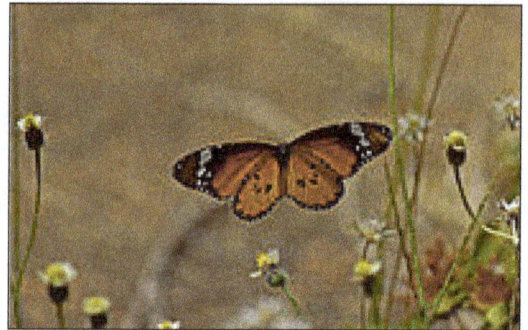

The Neoptera, including butterflies and most other insects, have indirect flight musculature.

Other than the two orders with direct flight muscles, all other living winged insects fly using a different mechanism, involving indirect flight muscles. This mechanism evolved once and is the defining feature (synapomorphy) for the infraclass Neoptera; it corresponds, probably not coincidentally, with the appearance of a wing-folding mechanism, which allows Neopteran insects to fold the wings back over the abdomen when at rest (though this ability has been lost secondarily in some groups, such as in the butterflies).

In the higher groups with two functional pairs of wings, both pairs are linked together mechanically in various ways and function as a single wing, although this is not true in the more primitive groups. There are also exceptions to be found among the more advanced Neoptera; the ghost moth is able to unlock its pair of wings and move them independently, allowing them to hover like dragonflies.

What all Neoptera share, however, is the way the muscles in the thorax work: these muscles, rather than attaching to the wings, attach to the thorax and deform it; since the wings are extensions of the thoracic exoskeleton, the deformations of the thorax cause the wings to move as well. A set of *dorsal longitudinal muscles* compresses the thorax from front to back, causing the dorsal surface of the thorax (notum) to bow upward, making the wings flip down. A set of *tergosternal muscles* pulls the notum downward again, causing the wings to flip upward. In a few groups, the downstroke is accomplished solely through the elastic recoil of the thorax when the tergosternal muscles are relaxed.

Several small sclerites at the wing base have other, separate, muscles attached and these are used for fine control of the wing base in such a way as to allow various adjustments in the tilt and amplitude of the wing beats.

Insects that beat their wings fewer than one hundred times a second use synchronous muscle. A synchronous muscle is a type of muscle that contracts once for every nerve impulse, which is more efficient for fast flight.

Insects that beat their wings more rapidly, such as the bumblebee, use asynchronous muscle; this is a type of muscle that contracts more than once per nerve impulse. This is achieved by the muscle being stimulated to contract again by a release in tension in the muscle, which can happen more rapidly than through simple nerve stimulation alone. This allows the frequency of wing beats to exceed the rate at which the nervous system can send impulses. The asynchronous muscle is one of the final refinements that has appeared in some of the higher Neoptera (Coleoptera, Diptera, and Hymenoptera). The overall effect is that many higher Neoptera can beat their wings much faster than insects with direct flight muscles.

Aerodynamics

There are two basic aerodynamic models of insect flight: creating a leading edge vortex, and using clap and fling.

Leading Edge Vortex

Most insects use a method that creates a spiralling leading edge vortex. These flapping wings move through two basic half-strokes. The downstroke starts up and back and is plunged downward and forward. Then the wing is quickly flipped over (supination) so that the leading edge is pointed backward. The upstroke then pushes the wing upward and backward. Then the wing is flipped again (pronation) and another downstroke can occur. The frequency range in insects with synchronous flight muscles typically is 5 to 200 hertz (Hz). In those with asynchronous flight muscles, wing beat frequency may exceed 1000 Hz. When the insect is hovering, the two strokes take the same amount of time. A slower downstroke, however, provides thrust.

Identification of major forces is critical to understanding insect flight. The first attempts to understand flapping wings assumed a quasi-steady state. This means that the air flow over the wing at any given time was assumed to be the same as how the flow would be over a non-flapping, steady-state wing at the same angle of attack. By dividing the flapping wing into a large number of motionless positions and then analyzing each position, it would be possible to create a timeline of the instantaneous forces on the wing at every moment. The calculated lift was found to be too small by a factor of three, so researchers realized that there must be unsteady phenomena providing aerodynamic forces. There were several developing analytical models attempting to approximate flow close to a flapping wing. Some researchers predicted force peaks at supination. With a dynamically scaled model of a fruit fly, these predicted forces later were confirmed. Others argued that the force peaks during supination and pronation are caused by an unknown rotational effect that fundamentally is different from the translational phenomena. There is some disagreement with this argument. Through computational fluid dynamics, some researchers argue that there is no rotational effect. They claim that the high forces are caused by an interaction with the wake shed by the previous stroke.

Similar to the rotational effect, the phenomena associated with flapping wings are not completely understood or agreed upon. Because every model is an approximation, different models leave out effects that are presumed to be negligible. For example, the Wagner effect says that circulation rises slowly to its steady-state due to viscosity when an inclined wing is accelerated from rest. This phenomenon would explain a lift value that is less than what is predicted. Typically, the case has been to find sources for the added lift. It has been argued that this effect is negligible for flow with a Reynolds number that is typical of insect flight. The Wagner effect was ignored, consciously, in at least one recent model. One of the most important phenomena that occurs during insect flight is leading edge suction. This force is significant to the calculation of efficiency. The concept of leading edge suction first was put forth to describe vortex lift on sharp-edged delta wings. At high angles of attack, the flow separates over the leading edge, but reattaches before reaching the trailing edge. Within this bubble of separated flow is a vortex. Because the angle of attack is so high, a lot of momentum is transferred downward into the flow. These two features create a large amount of lift force as well as some additional drag. The important feature, however, is the lift. Because the flow has separated, yet it still provides large amounts of lift, this phenomenon is called *stall delay*. This effect was observed in flapping insect flight and it was proven to be capable of providing enough lift to account for the deficiency in the quasi-steady-state models. This effect is used by canoeists in a sculling draw stroke.

All of the effects on a flapping wing may be reduced to three major sources of aerodynamic phenomena: the leading edge vortex, the steady-state aerodynamic forces on the wing, and the wing's contact with its wake from previous strokes. The size of flying insects ranges from about 20 micrograms to about 3 grams. As insect body mass increases, wing area increases and wing beat frequency decreases. For larger insects, the Reynolds number (Re) may be as high as 10000. For smaller insects, it may be as low as 10. This means that viscous effects are much more important to the smaller insects, although the flow is still laminar, even in the largest fliers.

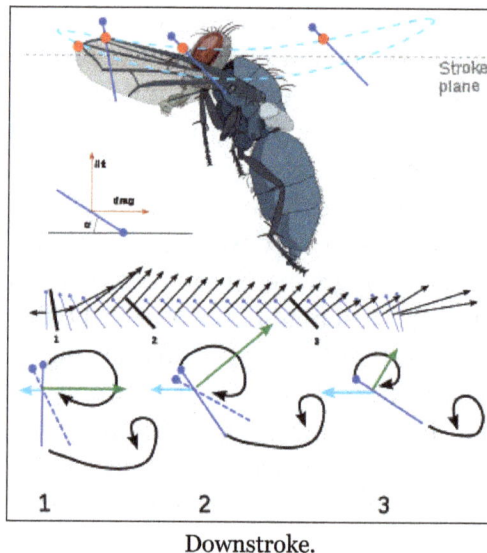

Downstroke.

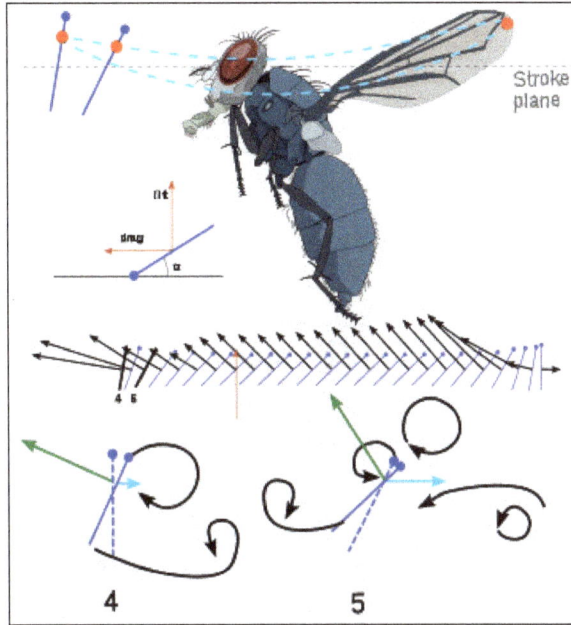

Upstroke.

Another interesting feature of insect flight is the body tilt. As flight speed increases, the insect body tends to tilt nose-down and become more horizontal. This reduces the frontal area and therefore, the body drag. Since drag also increases as forward velocity increases, the insect is making its flight more efficient as this efficiency becomes more necessary. Additionally, by changing the geometric angle of attack on the downstroke, the insect is able to keep its flight at an optimal efficiency through as many manoeuvres as possible. The development of general thrust is relatively small compared with lift forces. Lift forces may be more than three times the insect's weight, while thrust at even the highest speeds may be as low as 20% of the weight. This force is developed primarily through the less powerful upstroke of the flapping motion.

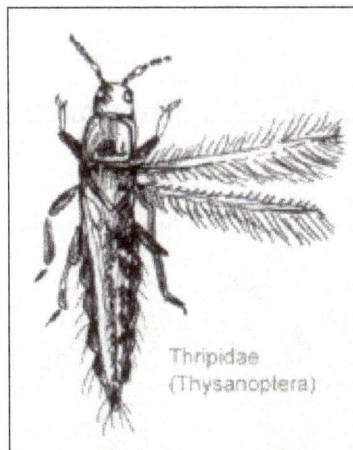

The feathery wings of a thrips are unsuitable for the leading edge
vortex flight of most other insects, but support clap and fling flight.

Clap and Fling

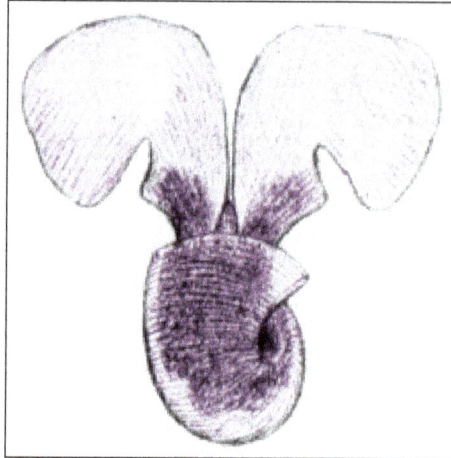

Clap and fling is used in sea butterflies such as
Limacina helicina to "fly" through the water.

The second method of flight, clap and fling, or the Weis-Fogh mechanism, functions differently. In this process, found in very small insects such as thrips and chalcid wasps, the wings clap together above the insect's body and then fling apart. As they fling open, the air gets sucked in and creates a vortex over each wing. This bound vortex then moves across the wing and, in the clap, acts as the starting vortex for the other wing. By this effect, circulation and thus lift are increased to the extent of being higher, in most cases, than the typical leading edge vortex effect. One of the reasons this method is not employed by more insects is the inevitable damage and wear to the wings caused by repeated clapping. It is prevalent, however, among insects that are very small and experience low Reynolds numbers. The mechanism is also employed by the marine mollusc *Limacina helicina*, a sea butterfly. Some insects, such as the vegetable leaf miner *Liriomyza sativae*, exploit a partial clap and fling, using the mechanism only on the outer part of the wing to increase lift by some 7% when hovering.

Clap and Fling Flight Mechanism after Sane 2003

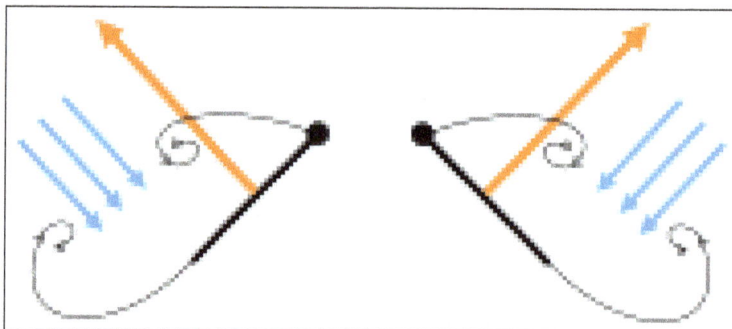

Wings close over back.

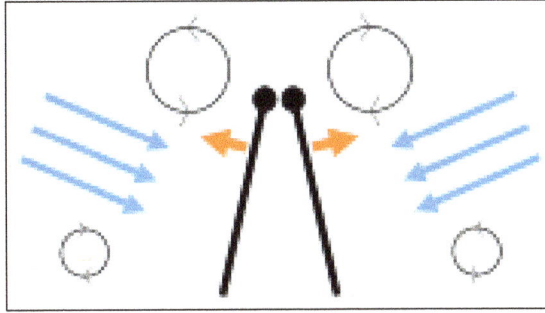

Leading edges touch, wing rotates around leading edge, vortices form.

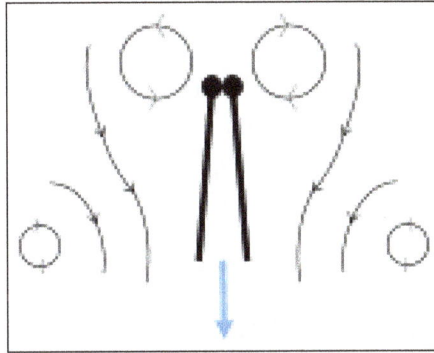

Trailing edges close, vortices shed, wings close giving thrust.

Black (Curved) Arrows: Flow; Blue Arrows: Induced Velocity; Orange Arrows: Net Force on Wing.

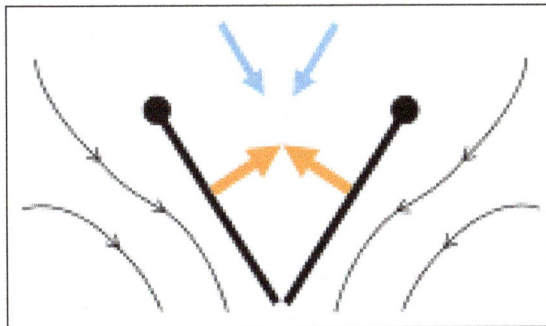

Wings rotate around trailing edge to fling apart.

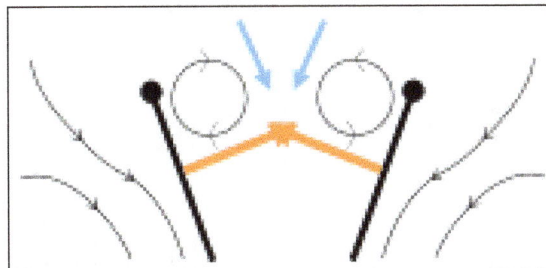

Leading edge moves away, air rushes in, increasing lift.

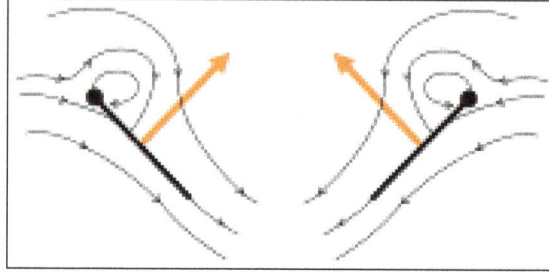

New vortex forms at leading edge, trailing edge vortices cancel each
other, perhaps helping flow to grow faster.

Governing Equations

A wing moving in fluids experiences a fluid force, which follows the conventions found in aerodynamics. The force component normal to the direction of the far field flow relative to the wing is referred to as lift (L), and the force component in the opposite direction of the flow is drag (D). At the Reynolds numbers considered here, an appropriate force unit is $1/2(\rho U^2 S)$, where ρ is the density of the fluid, S the wing area, and U the wing speed. The dimensionless forces are called lift (C_L) and drag (C_D) coefficients, that is:

$$C_L(\alpha) = \frac{2L}{\rho U^2 S} \quad \text{and} \quad C_D(\alpha) = \frac{2D}{\rho U^2 S}.$$

C_L and C_D are constants only if the flow is steady. A special class of objects such as airfoils may reach a steady state when it slices through the fluid at a small angle of attack. In this case, the inviscid flow around an airfoil can be approximated by a potential flow satisfying the no-penetration boundary condition. The Kutta-Joukowski theorem of a 2D airfoil further assumes that the flow leaves the sharp trailing edge smoothly, and this determines the total circulation around an airfoil. The corresponding lift is given by Bernoulli's principle (Blasius theorem):

$$C_L = 2\pi \sin\alpha \quad \text{and} \quad C_D = 0.$$

The flows around birds and insects can be considered incompressible: The Mach number, or speed while moving through air, is typically 1/300 and the wing frequency is about 10–103 Hz. Using the governing equation as the Navier-Stokes equation being subject to the no-slip boundary condition, the equation is:

$$\frac{\partial u}{\partial t} + \left(u \cdot \nabla\right)u = -\frac{\nabla p}{\rho} + v\nabla^2 u$$

$$\nabla \cdot u = 0$$

$$u_{bd} = u_s.$$

Where u(x, t) is the flow field, p the pressure, ρ the density of the fluid, v the kinematic viscosity, ubd the velocity at the boundary, and us the velocity of the solid. By choosing a length scale, L, and velocity scale, U, the equation can be expressed in nondimensional form containing the Reynolds number, Re=UL/v . There are two obvious differences between an insect wing and an airfoil: An insect wing is much smaller and it flaps. Using a dragonfly as an example, Its chord (c) is about 1 cm, its wing length (l) about 4 cm, and its wing frequency (f) about 40 Hz. The tip speed (u) is about 1 m/s, and the corresponding Reynolds number, Re=uc/v about 103. At the smaller end, a Chalcid wasp has a wing length of about 0.5–0.7 mm and beats its wing at about 400 Hz. Its Reynolds number is about 25. The range of Reynolds number in insect flight is about 10 to 10^4, which lies in between the two limits that are convenient for theories: inviscid steady flows around an airfoil and Stokes flow experienced by a swimming bacterium. For this reason, this intermediate range is not well understood. On the other hand, it is perhaps the most ubiquitous regime among the things we see. Falling leaves and seeds, fishes, and birds all encounter unsteady flows similar to that seen around an insect.

In addition to the Reynolds number, there are at least two other relevant dimensionless parameters. A wing has three velocity scales: the flapping velocity with respect to the body (u), the forward velocity of the body (U_o), and the pitching velocity (Ωc). The ratios of them form two dimensionless variables, U_o/u and $\Omega c/u$, the former is often referred to as the advance ratio, and it is also related to the reduced frequency, fc/U_o.

If an insect wing is rigid, for example, a *Drosophila* wing is approximately so, its motion relative to a fixed body can be described by three variables: the position of the tip in spherical coordinates, ($\Theta(t),\Phi(t)$), and the pitching angle $\psi(t)$, about the axis connecting the root and the tip. To estimate the aerodynamic forces based on blade-element analysis, it is also necessary to determine the angle of attack (α). The typical angle of attack at 70% wingspan ranges from 25° to 45° in hovering insects (15° in hummingbirds). Despite the wealth of data available for many insects, relatively few experiments report the time variation of α during a stroke. They include wind tunnel experiments of a tethered locust and a tethered fly, and free hovering flight of a fruit fly.

Because they are relatively easy to measure, the wing-tip trajectories have been reported more frequently. For example, selecting only flight sequences that produced enough lift to support a weight, will show that the wing tip follows an elliptical shape. Non-crossing shapes were also reported for other insects. Regardless of their exact shapes, the plugging-down motion indicates that insects may use aerodynamic drag in addition to lift to support its weight.

Hovering

Flight parameters	Speed/mph	Beats/s
Aeshnid dragonfly	15.6	38
Hornet	12.8	100
Hummingbird hawkmoth	11.1	85
Horsefly	8.8	96

Syrphid hoverfly	7.8	120
Bumblebee	6.4	130
Honeybee	5.7	250
Housefly	4.4	190
Damselfly	3.3	16
Scorpionfly	1.1	28
Large white butterfly	5.6	12
Thrips (clap and fling)	0.68	254

Many insects can hover, or stay in one spot in the air, doing so by beating their wings rapidly. The ability to do so, though, is complex; requiring the use of sideways stabilization as well as the lift necessary to overcome the force of gravity. The lifting force is caused by the downward stroke of the wings. As the wings push down on the surrounding air, the result reaction force of the air on the wings force the insect up. The wings of most insects are evolved so that, during the upward stroke, the force on the wing is small. Due to the fact that the upbeat and downbeat force the insect down and up respectively, the insect oscillates and winds up staying in the same position.

The distance the insect falls between wingbeats depends on how rapidly its wings are beating. If the insect flaps its wings at a slow rate, the time interval during which the lifting force is zero is longer, and therefore the insect falls farther than if its wings were beating rapidly. One can calculate the wingbeat frequency necessary for the insect to maintain a given stability in its amplitude. To simplify the calculations, one must assume that the lifting force is at a finite constant value while the wings are moving down and that it is zero while the wings are moving up. During the time interval Δt of the upward wingbeat, the insect drops a distance h under the influence of gravity.

$$h = \frac{g(\Delta t^2)}{2}$$

The upward stroke then restores the insect to its original position. Typically, it may be required that the vertical position of the insect change by no more than 0.1 mm (i.e., h=0.1 mm). The maximum allowable time for free fall is then:

$$\Delta t = \left(\frac{2h}{g}\right)^{1/2} = \sqrt{\frac{2 \times 10^{-2} \text{ cm}}{980 \text{ cm}/\text{s}^2}} \approx 4.5 \times 10^{-3} \text{ s}$$

Since the up movements and the down movements of the wings are about equal in duration, the period T for a complete up-and-down wing is twice Δr, that is,

$$T = 2\Delta t = 9 \times 10^{-3} \text{ s}$$

The frequency of the beats, f, meaning the number of wingbeats per second, is represented by the equation:

$$f = \frac{1}{T} \approx 110 \text{ s}^{-1}$$

In the examples used the frequency used is 110 beats/s, which is the typical frequency found in insects. Butterflies have a much slower frequency with about 10 beats/s, which means that they can't hover. Other insects may be able to produce a frequency of 1000 beats/s. To restore the insect to its original vertical position, the average upward force during the downward stroke, F_{av}, must be equal to twice the weight of the insect. Note that since the upward force on the insect body is applied only for half the time, the average upward force on the insect is simply its weight.

Power Input

One can now compute the power required to maintain hovering by, considering again an insect with mass m 0.1 g, average force, F_{av}, applied by the two wings during the downward stroke is two times the weight. Because the pressure applied by the wings is uniformly distributed over the total wing area, that means one can assume the force generated by each wing acts through a single point at the midsection of the wings. During the downward stroke, the center of the wings traverses a vertical distance d. The total work done by the insect during each downward stroke is the product of force and distance; that is,

$$\text{Work} = F_{av} \times d = 2\text{Wd}$$

If the wings swing through the beat at an angle of 70°, then in the case presented for the insect with 1 cm long wings, d is 0.57 cm. Therefore, the work done during each stroke by the two wings is:

$$\text{Work} = 2 \times 0.1 \times 980 \times 0.57 = 112 \text{erg}$$

After, the energy has to go somewhere; here, in the example used, the mass of the insect has to be raised 0.1 mm during each downstroke. The energy E required for this task is:

$$E = \text{mgh} = 0.1 \times 980 \times 10^{-2} = 0.98 \text{erg}$$

This is a negligible fraction of the total energy expended which clearly, most of the energy is expended in other processes. A more detailed analysis of the problem shows that the work done by the wings is converted primarily into kinetic energy of the air that is accelerated by the downward stroke of the wings. The power is the amount of work done in 1 s; in the insect used as an example, makes 110 downward strokes per second. Therefore, its power output P is, strokes per second, and that means its power output P is:

$$P = 112 \text{erg} \times 110/\text{s} = 1.23 \times 10^4 \text{erg/s} = 1.23 \times 10^{-3} \text{W}$$

Power Output

In the calculation of the power used in hovering, the examples used neglected the kinetic energy of the moving wings. The wings of insects, light as they are, have a finite mass; therefore, as they move they possess kinetic energy. Because the wings are in rotary motion, the maximum kinetic energy during each wing stroke is:

$$KE = \frac{1}{2} I \omega_{max}^2$$

Here I is the moment of inertia of the wing and ω_{max} is the maximum angular velocity during the wing stroke. To obtain the moment of inertia for the wing, we will assume that the wing can be approximated by a thin rod pivoted at one end. The moment of inertia for the wing is then:

$$I = \frac{m\ell^2}{3}$$

Where l is the length of the wing (1 cm) and m is the mass of two wings, which may be typically 10^{-3} g. The maximum angular velocity, ω_{max}, can be calculated from the maximum linear velocity, v_{max}, at the center of the wing:

$$\omega_{max} = \frac{v_{max}}{\ell/2}$$

During each stroke the center of the wings moves with an average linear velocity v_{av} given by the distance d traversed by the center of the wing divided by the duration Δt of the wing stroke. From our previous example, d=0.57 cm and $\Delta t = 4.5 \times 10^{-3}$ s. Therefore:

$$v_{av} = \frac{d}{\Delta t} = \frac{0.57}{4.5 \times 10^{-3}} = 127 \text{cm/s}$$

The velocity of the wings is zero both at the beginning and at the end of the wing stroke, meaning the maximum linear velocity is higher than the average velocity. If we assume that the velocity varies sinusoidally along the wing path, the maximum velocity is twice as high as the average velocity. Therefore, the maximum angular velocity is:

$$\omega_{max} = \frac{254}{\ell/2}$$

And the kinetic energy therefore is:

$$KE = \frac{1}{2}I\omega_{max}^2 = \left(10^{-3}\frac{\ell^2}{3}\right)\left(\frac{254}{\ell/2}\right)^2 = 43 \text{ erg}$$

Since there are two wing strokes (the upstroke and downstroke) in each cycle of the wing movement, the kinetic energy is 2×43=86 erg. This is about as much energy as is consumed in hovering itself.

Elasticity

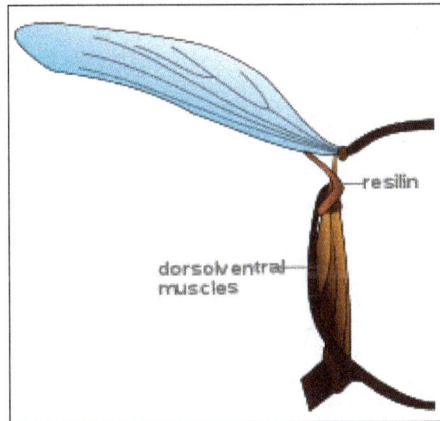

Insects gain kinetic energy, provided by the muscles, when they accelerate. When the wings begin to decelerate toward the end of the stroke, this energy must dissipate. During the downstroke, the kinetic energy is dissipated by the muscles themselves and is converted into heat (this heat is sometimes used to maintain core body temperature). Some insects are able to utilize the kinetic energy in the upward movement of the wings to aid in their flight. The wing joints of these insects contain a pad of elastic, rubber-like protein called resilin. During the upstroke of the wing, the resilin is stretched. The kinetic energy of the wing is converted into potential energy in the stretched resilin, which stores the energy much like a spring. When the wing moves down, this energy is released and aids in the downstroke.

Using a few simplifying assumptions, we can calculate the amount of energy stored in the stretched resilin. Although the resilin is bent into a complex shape, the example given shows the calculation as a straight rod of area A and length. Furthermore, we will assume that throughout the stretch the resilin obeys Hooke's law. This is not strictly true as the resilin is stretched by a considerable amount and therefore both the area and Young's modulus change in the process of stretching. The energy E stored in the stretched resilin is:

$$E = \frac{1}{2}\frac{YA\Delta\ell^2}{\ell}$$

Here Y is the Young's modulus for resilin, which has been measured to be 1.8×10^7 dyn/cm². Typically, in an insect the size of a bee the volume of the resilin may be equivalent to a cylinder 2×10^{-2} cm long and 4×10^{-4} cm² in area. In the example given, the length of the resilin rod is increased by 50% when stretched. That is, $\Delta\ell$ is 10^{-2} cm. Therefore, in this case the energy stored in the resilin of each wing is:

$$E = \frac{1}{2} \frac{1.8 \times 10^7 \times 4 \times 10^{-4} \times 10^{-4}}{2 \times 10^{-2}} = 18 \text{ erg}$$

The stored energy in the two wings is 36 erg, which is comparable to the kinetic energy in the upstroke of the wings. Experiments show that as much as 80% of the kinetic energy of the wing may be stored in the resilin.

Wing Coupling

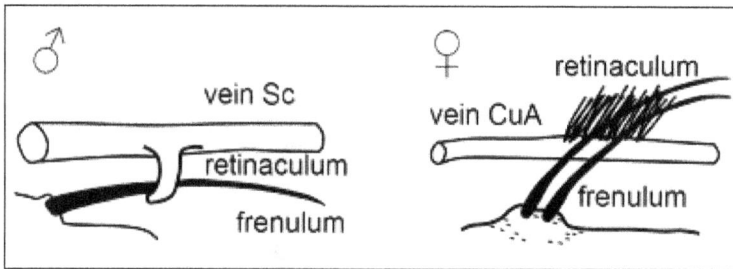

Frenulo-retinacular wing coupling in male and female moths.

Some four-winged insect orders, such as the Lepidoptera, have developed a wide variety of morphological wing coupling mechanisms in the imago which render these taxa as "functionally dipterous". All but the most basal forms exhibit this wing-coupling.

The mechanisms are of three different types - jugal, frenulo-retinacular and amplexiform.

The more primitive groups have an enlarged lobe-like area near the basal posterior margin, i.e. at the base of the forewing, called *jugum*, that folds under the hindwing in flight.

Other groups have a frenulum on the hindwing that hooks under a retinaculum on the forewing.

In the butterflies (except the male of one species of hesperiid) and in the Bombycoidea (except the Sphingidae), there is no arrangement of frenulum and retinaculum to couple the wings. Instead, an enlarged humeral area of the hindwing is broadly overlapped by the forewing. Despite the absence of a specific mechanical connection, the wings overlap and operate in phase. The power stroke of the forewing pushes down the hindwing in unison. This type of coupling is a variation of frenate type but where the frenulum and retinaculum are completely lost.

Biochemistry

The biochemistry of insect flight has been a focus of considerable study. While many insects use carbohydrates and lipids as the energy source for flight, many beetles and flies use the amino acid proline as their energy source. Some species also use a combination of sources and moths such as *Manduca sexta* use carbohydrates for pre-flight warm-up.

AQUATIC LOCOMOTION

Aquatic locomotion is biologically propelled motion through a liquid medium. The simplest propulsive systems are composed of cilia and flagella. Swimming has evolved a number of times in a range of organisms including arthropods, fish, molluscs, reptiles, birds, and mammals.

Micro-organisms

Ciliates

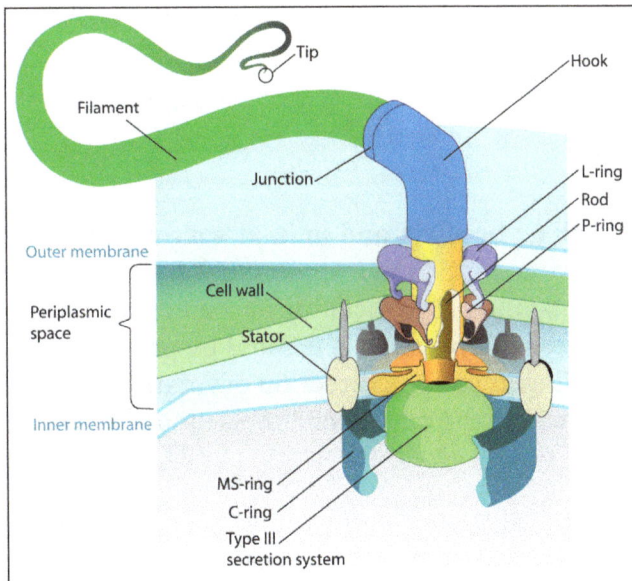

The flagellum of a Gram-negative bacteria
is rotated by a molecular motor at its base.

Ciliates use small flagella called cilia to move through the water. One ciliate will generally have hundreds to thousands of cilia that are densely packed together in arrays. During movement, an individual cilium deforms using a high-friction power stroke followed by a low-friction recovery stroke. Since there are multiple cilia packed together on an individual organism, they display collective behavior in a metachronal rhythm. This means the deformation of one cilium is in phase with the deformation of its neighbor, causing deformation waves that propagate along the surface of the organism. These propagating waves of cilia are what allow the organism to use the cilia in a coordinated manner to move. A typical example of a ciliated microorganism is the *Paramecium*, a one-celled, ciliated protozoan covered by thousands of cilia. The cilia beating together allow the *Paramecium* to propel through the water at speeds of 500 micrometers per second.

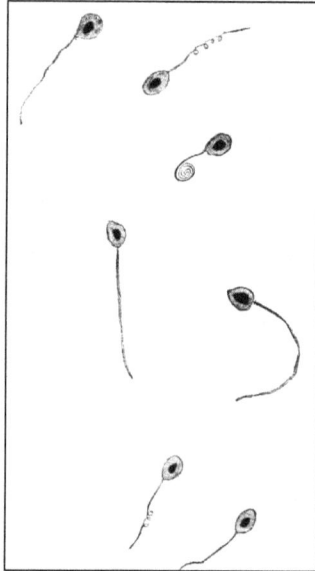

Salmon spermatozoa for artificial propagation.

Flagellates

Certain organisms such as bacteria and animal sperm have flagellum which have developed a way to move in liquid environments. A rotary motor model shows that bacteria uses the protons of an electrochemical gradient in order to move their flagella. Torque in the flagella of bacteria is created by particles that conduct protons around the base of the flagellum. The direction of rotation of the flagella in bacteria comes from the occupancy of the proton channels along the perimeter of the flagellar motor.

Movement of sperm is called sperm motility. The middle of the mammalian spermatozoon contains mitochondria that power the movement of the flagellum of the sperm. The motor around the base produces torque, just like in bacteria for movement through the aqueous environment.

Pseudopodia

Movement using a pseudopod is accomplished through increases in pressure at one point on the cell membrane. This pressure increase is the result of actin polymerization between the cortex and the membrane. As the pressure increases the cell membrane is pushed outward creating the pseudopod. When the pseudopod moves outward, the rest of the body is pulled forward by cortical tension. The result is cell movement through the fluid medium. Furthermore, the direction of movement is determined by chemotaxis. When chemoattraction occurs in a particular area of the cell membrane, actin polymerization can begin and move the cell in that direction. An excellent example of an organism that utilizes pseudopods is *Naegleria fowleri*.

Invertebrates

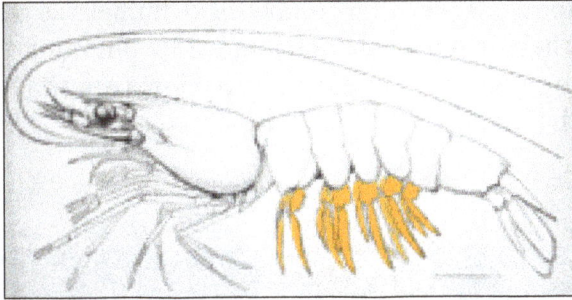

Shrimp paddle with special swimming legs (pleopods).

Among the radiata, jellyfish and their kin, the main form of swimming is to flex their cup shaped bodies. All jellyfish are free-swimming, although many of these spend most of their time swimming passively. Passive swimming is akin to gliding; the organism floats, using currents where it can, and does not exert any energy into controlling its position or motion. Active swimming, in contrast, involves the expenditure of energy to travel to a desired location.

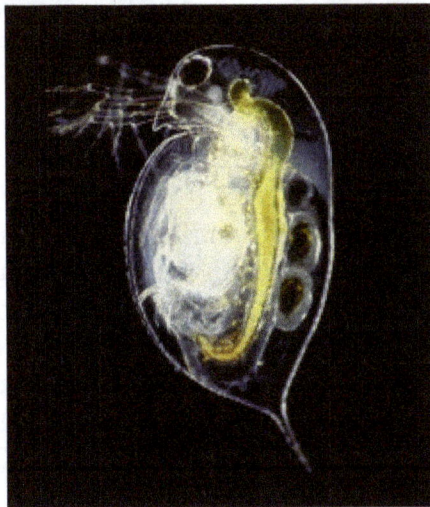

Daphnia swims by beating its antennae.

In bilateria, there are many methods of swimming. The arrow worms (chaetognatha) undulate their finned bodies, not unlike fish. Nematodes swim by undulating their fin-less bodies. Some Arthropod groups can swim - including many crustaceans. Most crustaceans, such as shrimp, will usually swim by paddling with special swimming legs (pleopods). Swimming crabs swim with modified walking legs (pereiopods). Daphnia, a crustacean, swims by beating its antennae instead.

There are also a number of forms of swimming molluscs. Many free-swimming sea slugs, such as sea angels, flap fin-like structures. Some shelled molluscs, such as scallops can briefly swim by clapping their two shells open and closed. The molluscs most evolved for swimming are the cephalopods.

Among the Deuterostomia, there are a number of swimmers as well. Feather stars can swim by undulating their many arms. Salps move by pumping waters through their gelatinous bodies. The deuterostomes most evolved for swimming are found among the vertebrates, notably the fish.

Jet Propulsion

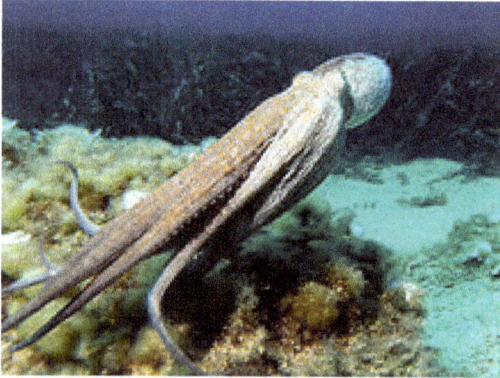

Octopuses swim headfirst, with arms trailing behind.

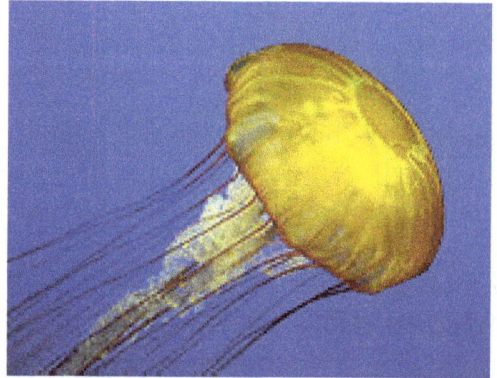

Jellyfish pulsate their bell for a type of jet locomotion.

Jet propulsion is a method of aquatic locomotion where animals fill a muscular cavity and squirt out water to propel them in the opposite direction of the squirting water. Most organisms are equipped with one of two designs for jet propulsion; they can draw water from the rear and expel it from the rear, such as jellyfish, or draw water from front and expel it from the rear, such as salps. Filling up the cavity causes an increase in both the mass and drag of the animal. Because of the expanse of the contracting cavity, the animal's velocity fluctuates as it moves through the water, accelerating while expelling water and decelerating while vacuuming water. Even though these fluctuations in drag and mass can be ignored if the frequency of the jet-propulsion cycles is high enough, jet-propulsion is a relatively inefficient method of aquatic locomotion.

All cephalopods can move by jet propulsion, but this is a very energy-consuming way to travel compared to the tail propulsion used by fish. The relative efficiency of jet propulsion decreases further as animal size increases. Since the Paleozoic, as competition with fish produced an environment where efficient motion was crucial to survival, jet propulsion has taken a back role, with fins and tentacles used to maintain a steady velocity. The stop-start motion provided by the jets, however, continues to be useful for providing bursts of high speed - not least when capturing prey or avoiding predators. Indeed, it makes cephalopods the fastest marine invertebrates, Preface and they can out accelerate most fish. Oxygenated water is taken into the mantle cavity to the gills and through muscular contraction of this cavity, the spent water is expelled through the hyponome, created by a fold in the mantle. Motion of the cephalopods is usually backward as water is forced out anteriorly through the hyponome, but direction can be controlled somewhat by pointing it in different directions. Most cephalopods float (i.e. are neutrally buoyant), so do not need to swim to remain afloat. Squid swim more slowly than fish, but use more power to generate their speed. The loss in efficiency is due to the amount of water the squid can accelerate out of its mantle cavity.

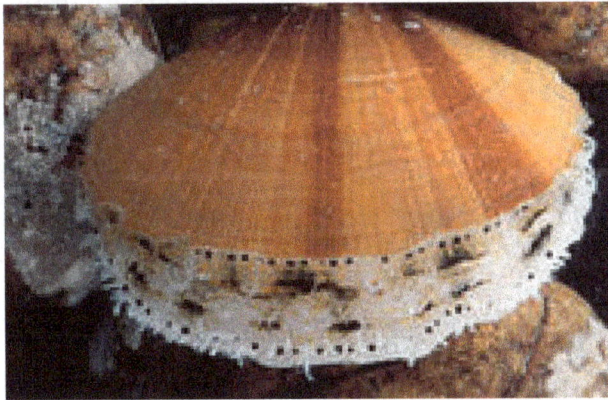

Scallops swim by clapping their two shells open and closed.

Jellyfish use a one-way water cavity design which generates a phase of continuous cycles of jet-propulsion followed by a rest phase. The Froude efficiency is about 0.09, which indicates a very costly method of locomotion. The metabolic cost of transport for jellyfish is high when compared to a fish of equal mass.

Other jet-propelled animals have similar problems in efficiency. Scallops, which use a similar design to jellyfish, swim by quickly opening and closing their shells, which draws in water and expels it from all sides. This locomotion is used as a means to escape predators such as starfish. Afterwards, the shell acts as a hydrofoil to counteract the scallop's tendency to sink. The Froude efficiency is low for this type of movement, about 0.3, which is why it's used as an emergency escape mechanism from predators. However, the amount of work the scallop has to do is mitigated by the elastic hinge that connects the two shells of the bivalve. Squids swim by drawing water into their mantle cavity and expelling it through their siphon. The Froude efficiency of their jet-propulsion system is around 0.29, which is much lower than a fish of the same mass.

Much of the work done by scallop muscles to close its shell is stored as elastic energy in abductin tissue, which acts as a spring to open the shell. The elasticity causes the work done against the water to be low because of the large openings the water has to enter and the small openings the water has to leave. The inertial work of scallop jet-propulsion is also low. Because of the low inertial work, the energy savings created by the elastic tissue is so small that it's negligible. Medusae can also use their elastic mesoglea to enlarge their bell. Their mantle contains a layer of muscle sandwiched between elastic fibers. The muscle fibers run around the bell circumferentially while the elastic fibers run through the muscle and along the sides of the bell to prevent lengthening. After making a single contraction, the bell vibrates passively at the resonant frequency to refill the bell. However, in contrast with scallops, the inertial work is similar to the hydrodynamic work due to how medusas expel water - through a large opening at low velocity. Because of this, the negative pressure created by the vibrating cavity is lower than the positive pressure of the jet, meaning that inertial work of the mantle is small. Thus, jet-propulsion is shown as an inefficient swimming technique.

Fish

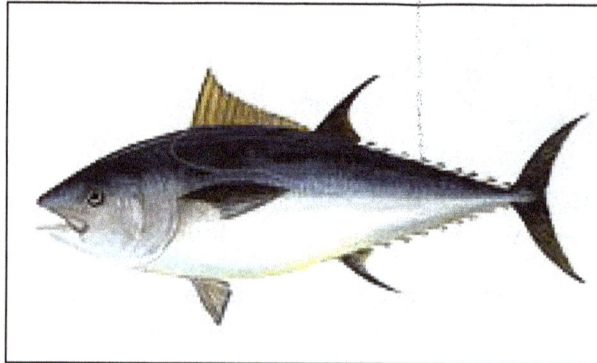

Open water fish, like this Atlantic bluefin tuna, are usually
streamlined for straightline speed, with a deeply forked tail
and a smooth body shaped like a spindle tapered at both ends.

Many fish swim through water by creating undulations with their bodies or oscillating their fins. The undulations create components of forward thrust complemented by a rearward force, side forces which are wasted portions of energy, and a normal force that is between the forward thrust and side force. Different fish swim by undulating different parts of their bodies. Eel-shaped fish undulate their entire body in rhythmic sequences. Streamlined fish, such as salmon, undulate the caudal portions of their bodies. Some fish, such as sharks, use stiff, strong fins to create dynamic lift and propel themselves. It is common for fish to use more than one form of propulsion, although they will display one dominant mode of swimming Gait changes have even been observed in juvenile reef fish of various sizes. Depending on their needs, fish can rapidly alternate between synchronized fin beats and alternating fin beats.

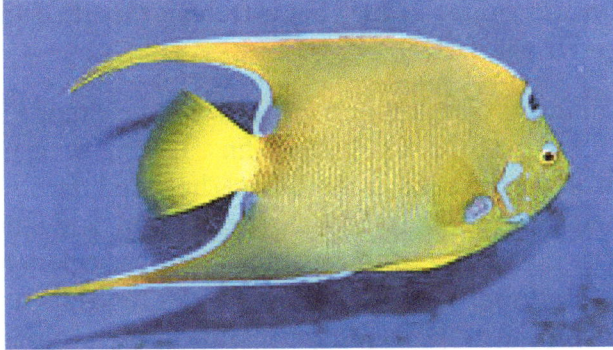
Many reef fish, like this queen angelfish, have a body
flattened like a pancake, with pectoral and pelvic fins that
act with the flattened body to maximize manoeuvrability.

According to *Guinness World Records 2009*, *Hippocampus zosterae* (the dwarf
seahorse) is the slowest moving fish, with a top speed of about 5 feet (150 cm) per hour.
They swim very poorly, rapidly fluttering a dorsal fin and using pectoral fins (located
behind their eyes) to steer. Seahorses have no caudal fin.

Body-caudal Fin (BCF) Propulsion

- Anguilliform: Anguilliform swimmers are typically slow swimmers. They undulate the majority of their body and use their head as the fulcrum for the load they are moving. At any point during their undulation, their body has an amplitude between 0.5-1.0 wavelengths. The amplitude that they move their body through allows them to swim backwards. Anguilliform locomotion is usually seen in fish with long, slender bodies like eels, lampreys, oarfish, and a number of catfish species.

- Subcarangiform, Carangiform, Thunniform: These swimmers undulate the posterior half of their body and are much faster than anguilliform swimmers. At any point while they are swimming, a wavelength <1 can be seen in the undulation pattern of the body. Some Carangiform swimmers include nurse sharks, bamboo sharks, and reef sharks. Thunniform swimmers are very fast and some common Thunniform swimmers include tuna, white sharks, salmon, jacks, and mako sharks. Thunniform swimmers only undulate their high aspect ratio caudal fin, so they are usually very stiff to push more water out of the way.

- Ostraciiform: Ostraciiform swimmers oscillate their caudal region, making them relatively slow swimmers. Boxfish, torpedo rays, and momyrs employ Ostraciiform locomotion. The cow fish uses Osctraciiform locomotion to hover in the water column.

Median Paired Fin (MPF) Propulsion

- Tetraodoniform, Balistiform, Diodontiform: These swimmers oscillate their median fins. They are typically slow swimmers, and some notable examples include the oceanic sunfish (which has extremely modified anal and dorsal fins), puffer fish, and triggerfish.

- Rajiform, Amiiform, Gymnotiform: This locomotory mode is accomplished by undulation of the pectoral and median fins. During their undulation pattern, a wavelength >1 can be seen in their fins. They are typically slow to moderate swimmers, and some examples include rays, bowfin, and knife fishes. The black ghost knife fish is a Gymnotiform swimmer that has a very long ventral ribbon fin. Thrust is produced by passing waves down the ribbon fin while the body remains rigid. This also allows the ghost knife fish to swim in reverse.

- Labriform: Labriform swimmers are also slow swimmers. They oscillate their pectoral fins to create thrust. Oscillating fins create thrust when a starting vortex is shed from the trailing edge of the fin. As the foil departs from the starting vortex, the effect of that vortex diminishes, while the bound circulation remains, producing lift. Labriform swimming can be viewed as continuously starting and stopping. Wrasses and surf perch are common Labriform swimmers.

Hydrofoils

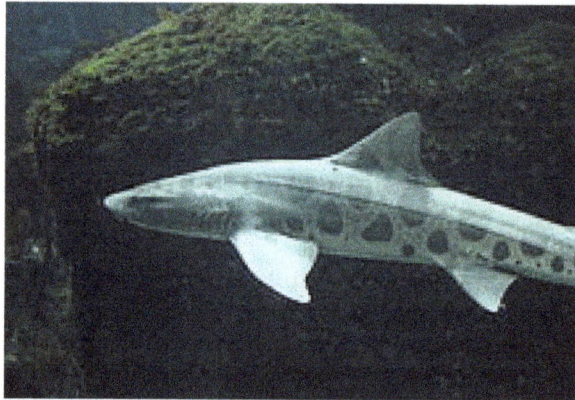

The leopard shark angles its pectoral fins so they
behave as hydrofoils to control the animal's pitch.

Hydrofoils, or fins, are used to push against the water to create a normal force to provide thrust, propelling the animal through water. Sea turtles and penguins beat their paired hydrofoils to create lift. Some paired fins, such as pectoral fins on leopard sharks, can be angled at varying degrees to allow the animal to rise, fall, or maintain its level in the water column. The reduction of fin surface area helps to minimize drag, and therefore increase efficiency. Regardless of size of the animal, at any particular speed, maximum possible lift is proportional to (wing area) x (speed)^2. Dolphins and whales have large, horizontal caudal hydrofoils, while many fish and sharks have vertical caudal hydrofoils. Porpoising (seen in cetaceans, penguins, and pinnipeds) may save energy if they are moving fast. Since drag increases with speed, the work required to swim unit distance is greater at higher speeds, but the work needed to jump unit distance is independent of speed. Seals propel themselves through the water with their caudal tail, while sea lions create thrust solely with their pectoral flippers.

Drag Powered Swimming

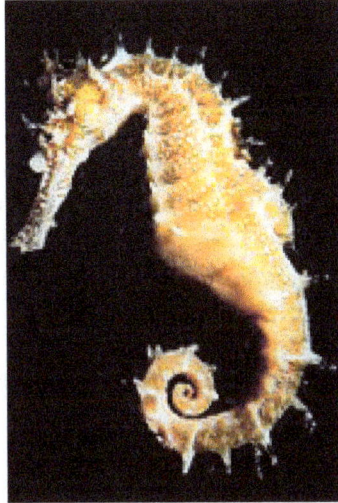

The slowest-moving fishes are the
sea horses, often found in reefs.

As with moving through any fluid, friction is created when molecules of the fluid collide with organism. The collision causes drag against moving fish, which is why many fish are streamlined in shape. Streamlined shapes work to reduce drag by orienting elongated objects parallel to the force of drag, therefore allowing the current to pass over and taper off the end of the fish. This streamlined shape allows for more efficient use of energy locomotion. Some flat-shaped fish can take advantage of pressure drag by having a flat bottom surface and curved top surface. The pressure drag created allows for the upward lift of the fish.

Appendages of aquatic organisms propel them in two main and biomechanically extreme mechanisms. Some use lift powered swimming, which can be compared to flying as appendages flap like wings, and reduce drag on the surface of the appendage. Others use drag powered swimming, which can be compared to oars rowing a boat, with movement in a horizontal plane, or paddling, with movement in the parasagittal plane.

Drag swimmers use a cyclic motion where they push water back in a power stroke, and return their limb forward in the return or recovery stroke. When they push water directly backwards, this moves their body forward, but as they return their limbs to the starting position, they push water forward, which will thus pull them back to some degree, and so opposes the direction that the body is heading. This opposing force is called drag. The return-stroke drag causes drag swimmers to employ different strategies than lift swimmers. Reducing drag on the return stroke is essential for optimizing efficiency. For example, ducks paddle through the water spreading the webs of their feet as they move water back, and then when they return their feet to the front they pull their webs together to reduce the subsequent pull of water forward. The legs of water beetles have little hairs which spread out to catch up and move water back in the power stroke, but lay flat as the appendage moves forward in the return stroke. Also, the water beetle's legs have a side that is wider and is held perpendicular to the motion when pushing backward, but the leg is then rotated when the limb is to return forward, so that the thinner side will catch up less water.

Drag swimmers experience a lessened efficiency in swimming due to resistance which affects their optimum speed. The less drag a fish experiences, the more it will be able to maintain higher speeds. Morphology of the fish can be designed to reduce drag, such as streamlining the body. The cost of transport is much higher for the drag swimmer, and when deviating from its optimum speed, the drag swimmer is energetically strained much more than the lift swimmer. There are natural processes in place to optimize energy use, and it is thought that adjustments of metabolic rates can compensate in part for mechanical disadvantages.

Semi-aquatic animals compared to fully aquatic animals exhibit exacerbation of drag. Design that allows them to function out of the water limits the efficiency possible to be reached when in the water. In water swimming at the surface exposes them to resistive wave drag and is associated with a higher cost than submerged swimming. Swimming below the surface exposes them to resistance due to return strokes and pressure, but primarily friction. Frictional drag is due to fluid viscosity and morphology characteristics. Pressure drag is due to the difference of water flow around the body and is also affected by body morphology. Semi-aquatic organisms encounter increased resistive forces when in or out of the water, as they are not specialized for either habitat. The morphology of otters and beavers, for example, must meet needs for both environments. Their fur decreases streamlining and creates additional drag. The platypus may be a good example of an intermediate between drag and lift swimmers because it has been shown to have a rowing mechanism which is similar to lift-based pectoral oscillation. The limbs of semi-aquatic organisms are reserved for use on land and using them in water not only increases the cost of locomotion, but limits them to drag-based modes. Although they are less efficient, drag swimmers are able to produce more thrust at low speeds than lift swimmers. They are also thought to be better for maneuverability due to the large thrust produced.

Amphibians

Most of the Amphibia have a larval state, which has inherited anguilliform motion, and a laterally compressed tail to go with it, from fish ancestors. The corresponding tetrapod adult forms, even in the tail-retaining sub-class Urodeles, are sometimes aquatic to only a negligible extent (as in the genus Salamandra, whose tail has lost its suitability for aquatic propulsion), but the majority of Urodeles, from the newts to the giant salamander Megalobatrachus, retain a laterally compressed tail for a life that is aquatic to a considerable degree, which can use in a carangiform motion.

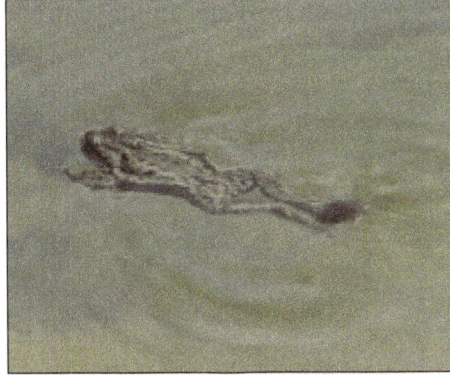

Common toad (Bufo bufo) swimming.

Of the tailless amphibians (the frogs and toads of the sub-class Anura) the majority are aquatic to an insignificant extent in adult life, but in that considerable minority that are mainly aquatic we encounter for the first time the problem of adapting the tailless-tetrapod structure for aquatic propulsion. The mode that they use is unrelated to any used by fish. With their flexible back legs and webbed feet they execute something close to the leg movements of a human 'breast stroke,' rather more efficiently because the legs are better streamlined.

Reptiles

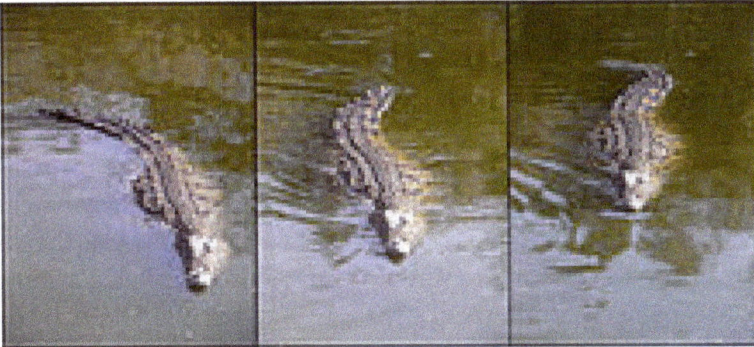

Nile crocodile (Crocodylus niloticus) swimming.

From the point of view of aquatic propulsion, the descent of modern members of the class Reptilia from archaic tailed Amphibia is most obvious in the case of the order Crocodilia (crocodiles and alligators), which use their deep, laterally compressed tails in an essentially carangiform mode of propulsion.

Terrestrial snakes, in spite of their 'bad' hydromechanical shape with roughly circular cross-section and gradual posterior taper, swim fairly readily when required, by an anguilliform propulsion.

Cheloniidae (true turtles) have found a beautiful solution to the problem of tetrapod swimming through the development of their forelimbs into flippers of high-aspect-ratio wing shape, with which they imitate a bird's propulsive mode more accurately than do the eagle-rays themselves.

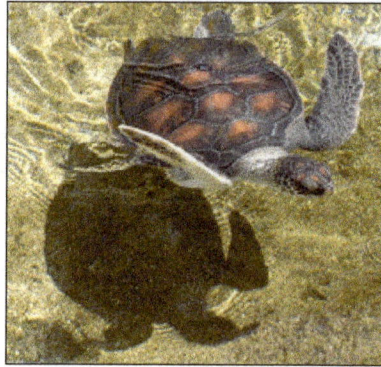
Immature Hawaiian green sea turtle in shallow waters.

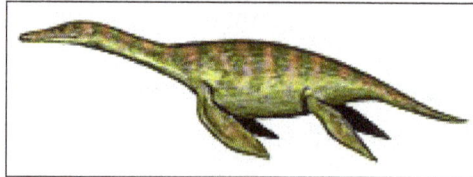
Macroplata.

Fin and Flipper Locomotion

Aquatic reptiles such as sea turtles and extinct species like Pliosauroids predominantly use their pectoral flippers to propel themselves through the water and their pelvic flippers for maneuvering. During swimming they move their pectoral flippers in a dorso-ventral motion, causing forward motion. During swimming, they rotate their front flippers to decrease drag through the water column and increase efficiency. Newly hatched sea turtles exhibit several behavioral skills that help orientate themselves towards the ocean as well as identifying the transition from sand to water. If rotated in the pitch, yaw or roll direction, the hatchlings are capable of counteracting the forces acting upon them by correcting with either their pectoral or pelvic flippers and redirecting themselves towards the open ocean.

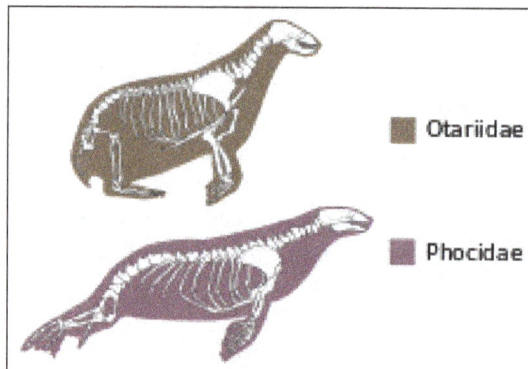

Otariidae

Phocidae

Comparative skeletal anatomy of a typical otariid seal and a typical phocid seal.

Among mammals otariids (fur seals) swim primarily with their front flippers, using the rear flippers for steering, and phocids (true seals) move the rear flippers laterally, pushing the animal through the water.

Escape Reactions

Some arthropods, such as lobsters and shrimps, can propel themselves backwards quickly by flicking their tail, known as lobstering or the caridoid escape reaction.

Varieties of fish, such as teleosts, also use fast-starts to escape from predators. Fast-starts are characterized by the muscle contraction on one side of the fish twisting the fish into a C-shape. Afterwards, muscle contraction occurs on the opposite side to allow the fish to enter into a steady swimming state with waves of undulation traveling alongside the body. The power of the bending motion comes from fast-twitch muscle fibers located in the central region of the fish. The signal to perform this contraction comes from a set of Mauthner cells which simultaneously send a signal to the muscles on one side of the fish. Mauthner cells are activated when something startles the fish and can be activated by visual or sound-based stimuli.

Fast-starts are split up into three stages. Stage one, which is called the preparatory stroke, is characterized by the initial bending to a C-shape with small delay caused by hydrodynamic resistance. Stage two, the propulsive stroke, involves the body bending rapidly to the other side, which may occur multiple times. Stage three, the rest phase, cause the fish to return to normal steady-state swimming and the body undulations begin to cease. Large muscles located closer to the central portion of the fish are stronger and generate more force than the muscles in the tail. This asymmetry in muscle composition causes body undulations that occur in Stage 3. Once the fast-start is completed, the position of the fish has been shown to have a certain level of unpredictability, which helps fish survive against predators.

The rate at which the body can bend is limited by resistance contained in the inertia of each body part. However, this inertia assists the fish in creating propulsion as a result of the momentum created against the water. The forward propulsion created from C-starts, and steady-state swimming in general, is a result of the body of the fish pushing against the water. Waves of undulation create rearward momentum against the water providing the forward thrust required to push the fish forward.

Efficiency

The Froude propulsion efficiency is defined as the ratio of power output to the power input:

$$nf = 2U_1 / (U_1 + U_2)$$

where U1 = free stream velocity and U2 = jet velocity. A good efficiency for carangiform propulsion is between 50 and 80%.

Minimizing Drag

Pressure differences occur outside the boundary layer of swimming organisms due to disrupted flow around the body. The difference on the up- and down-stream surfaces of the body is pressure drag, which creates a downstream force on the object. Frictional drag, on the other hand, is a result of fluid viscosity in the boundary layer. Higher turbulence causes greater frictional drag.

Reynolds number (Re) is the measure of the relationships between inertial and viscous forces in flow ((animal's length x animal's velocity)/kinematic viscosity of the fluid). Turbulent flow can be found at higher Re values, where the boundary layer separates and creates a wake, and laminar flow can be found at lower Re values, when the boundary layer separation is delayed, reducing wake and kinetic energy loss to opposing water momentum.

The body shape of a swimming organism affects the resulting drag. Long, slender bodies reduce pressure drag by streamlining, while short, round bodies reduce frictional drag; therefore, the optimal shape of an organism depends on its niche. Swimming organisms with a fusiform shape are likely to experience the greatest reduction in both pressure and frictional drag.

Wing shape also affects the amount of drag experienced by an organism, as with different methods of stroke, recovery of the pre-stroke position results in the accumulation of drag.

High-speed ram ventilation creates laminar flow of water from the gills along the body of an organism.

The secretion of mucus along the organism's body surface, or the addition of long-chained polymers to the velocity gradient, can reduce frictional drag experienced by the organism.

Buoyancy

Many aquatic/marine organisms have developed organs to compensate for their weight and control their buoyancy in the water. These structures, make the density of their bodies very close to that of the surrounding water. Some hydrozoans, such as siphonophores, has gas-filled floats; the Nautilus, Sepia, and Spirula (Cephalopods) have chambers of gas within their shells; and most teleost fish and many lantern fish (Myctophidae) are equipped with swim bladders. Many aquatic and marine organisms may also be composed of low-density materials. Deep-water teleosts, which do not have a swim bladder, have few lipids and proteins, deeply ossified bones, and watery tissues that maintain their buoyancy. Some sharks' livers are composed of low-density lipids, such as hydrocarbon squalene or wax esters (also found in Myctophidae without swim bladders), which provide buoyancy.

Swimming animals that are denser than water must generate lift or adapt a benthic lifestyle. Movement of the fish to generate hydrodynamic lift is necessary to prevent sinking. Often, their bodies act as hydrofoils, a task that is more effective in flat-bodied fish. At a small tilt angle, the lift is greater for flat fish than it is for fish with narrow bodies. Narrow-bodied fish use their fins as hydrofoils while their bodies remain horizontal. In sharks, the heterocercal tail shape drives water downward, creating a counteracting upward force while thrusting the shark forward. The lift generated is assisted by the pectoral fins and upward-angle body positioning. It is supposed that tunas primarily use their pectoral fins for lift.

Buoyancy maintenance is metabolically expensive. Growing and sustaining a buoyancy organ, adjusting the composition of biological makeup, and exerting physical strain to stay in motion demands large amounts of energy. It is proposed that lift may be physically generated at a lower energy cost by swimming upward and gliding downward, in a "climb and glide" motion, rather than constant swimming on a plane.

Temperature

Temperature can also greatly affect the ability of aquatic organisms to move through water. This is because temperature not only affects the properties of the water, but also the organisms in the water, as most have an ideal range specific to their body and metabolic needs.

Q10 (temperature coefficient), the factor by which a rate increases at a 10 °C increase in temperature, is used to measure how organisms' performance relies on temperature. Most have increased rates as water becomes warmer, but some have limits to this and others find ways to alter such effects, such as by endothermy or earlier recruitment of faster muscle.

For example, *Crocodylus porosus*, or estuarine crocodiles, were found to increase swimming speed from 15 °C to 23 °C and then to have peak swimming speed from 23 °C to 33 °C. However, performance began to decline as temperature rose beyond that point, showing a limit to the range of temperatures at which this species could ideally perform.

Submergence

The more of the animal's body that is submerged while swimming, the less energy it uses. Swimming on the surface requires two to three times more energy than when completely submerged. This is because of the bow wave that is formed at the front when the animal is pushing the surface of the water when swimming, creating extra drag.

TERRESTRIAL LOCOMOTION

Terrestrial locomotion is any of several forms of animal movement such as walking and running, jumping (saltation), and crawling. Walking and running, in which the body is carried well off the surface on which the animal is moving (substrate), occur only in arthropods and vertebrates. Running (cursorial) vertebrates are characterized by elongated lower legs and feet and by reduction and fusion of toes.

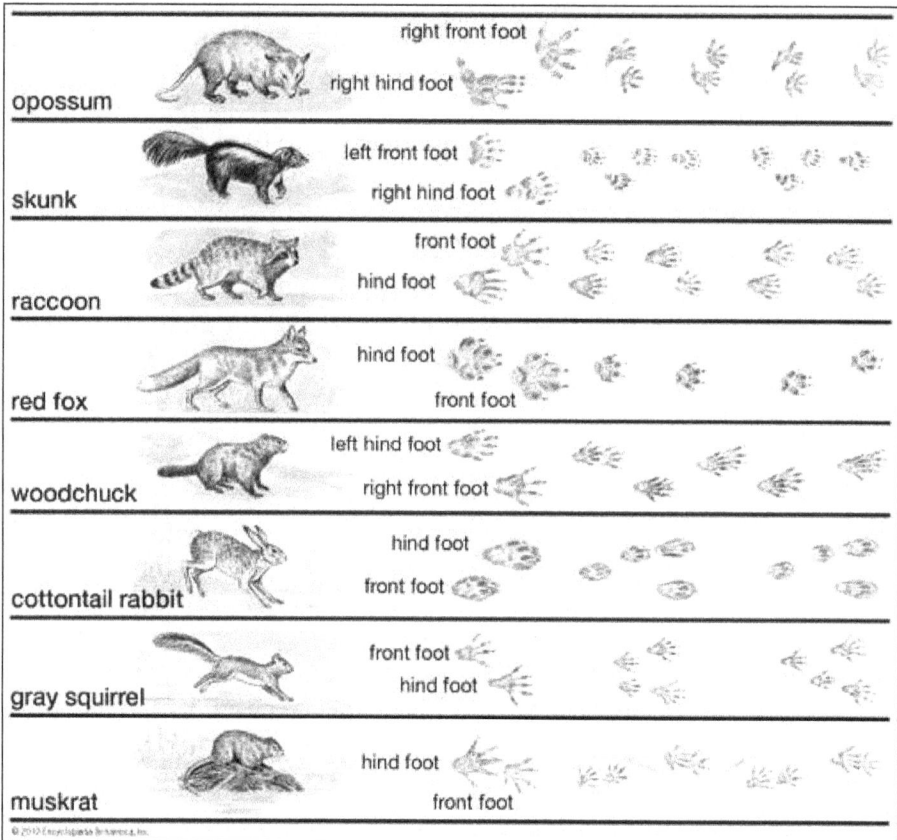

Animal tracks, Tracks of various North American mammals.

Saltatory locomotion, movement by leaping, hopping, or jumping, is found in a number of insects (e.g., fleas, grasshoppers) and vertebrates (frogs, kangaroos, rabbits and hares, some rodents). Specializations in mammalian saltators include, to varying degrees, enlargement of the hind legs and reduction of the forelegs; elongation of the midregion (metatarsals) of the hind foot; and elongation of the tail as a balancing organ.

Crawling differs from other forms of terrestrial locomotion in that the body touches or nearly touches the substrate. Many aquatic vertebrates, whose limbs are often short and poorly adapted for terrestrial movement, are restricted to crawling when on land. Snakes and other limbless vertebrates are highly adapted crawlers, using a variety of methods for gaining adhesion against the substrate.

References

- Locomotion, biology: byjus.com, Retrieved 09 May, 2019
- Difference-between-locomotion-and-movement, biology: byjus.com, Retrieved 15 August, 2019

- McNeill Alexander, R. (2002). Principles of Animal Locomotion. Princeton University Press. ISBN 978-0-691-08678-1

- Alexander, David E. Nature's Flyers: Birds, Insects, and the Biomechanics of Flight. 2002(hardcover) and 2004(paperback). Baltimore: The Johns Hopkins University Press. ISBN 0-8018-6756-8(hardcover) and 0801880599(paperback)

- Sane, Sanjay P. (2003). "The aerodynamics of insect flight" (PDF). The Journal of Experimental Biology. 206 (23): 4191–4208. doi:10.1242/jeb.00663. PMID 14581590

- Terrestrial-locomotion: britannica.com, Retrieved 14 March, 2019

6

Subfields of Biomechanics

The subfields of biomechanics include sports biomechanics, computational biomechanics, biofluid dynamics, nanobiomechanics, neuro biomechanics, kinesiology, biomechatronics, biotribology, etc. All these subfields of biomechanics have been carefully analyzed in this chapter.

SPORTS BIOMECHANICS

Biomechanics in sport incorporates a detailed analysis of sport movements in order to minimise the risk of injury and improve sports performance. Sport and exercise biomechanics encompasses the area of science concerned with the analysis of the mechanics of human movement. It refers to the description, detailed analysis and assessment of human movement during sport activities. Mechanics is a branch of physics that is concerned with the description of motion/movement and how forces create motion/movement. In other words, sport biomechanics is the science of explaining how and why the human body moves in the way that it does. In sport and exercise, that definition is often extended to also consider the interaction between the performer and their equipment and environment. Biomechanics is traditionally divided into the areas of kinematics which is a branch of mechanics that deals with the geometry of the motion of objects, including displacement, velocity, and acceleration, without taking into account the forces that produce the motion while kinetics is the study of the relationships between the force system acting on a body and the changes it produces in body motion. In terms of this, there are skeletal, muscular and neurological considerations we also need to consider when describing biomechanics.

Application

Human movement performance can be enhanced in many ways as effective movement encompasses anatomical factors, neuromuscular skills, physiological capacities and psychological/cognitive abilities. Biomechanics is essentially the science of movement technique and as such tends to be most utilised in sports where technique is a dominant factor rather than physical structure or physiological capacities. The following are some of the areas where biomechanics is applied, to either support the performance of athletes or solve issues in sport or exercise:

- The identification of optimal technique for enhancing sports performance.

- The analysis of body loading to determine the safest method for performing a particular sport or exercise task.

- The assessment of muscular recruitment and loading.

- The analysis of sport and exercise equipment e.g., shoes, surfaces and rackets.

Biomechanics is utilised to attempt to either enhance performance or reduce the injury risk in the sport and exercise tasks examined.

Principles of Biomechanics

It is important to know several biomechanical terms and principles when examining the role of biomechanics in sport and exercise.

Forces and Torques

A force is simply a push or pull and it changes the motion of a body segment or the racket. Motion is created and modified by the actions of forces (mostly muscle forces, but also by external forces from the environment). When force rotates a body segment or the racquet, this effect is called a torque or moment of force. Example - Muscles create a torque to rotate the body segments in all tennis strokes. In the service action internal rotation of the upper arm, so important to the power of the serve, is the result of an internal rotation torque at the shoulder joint caused by muscle actions (latissimus dorsi and parts of the pectoralis major and deltoid). To rotate a segment with more power a player would generally apply more muscle force.

Newton's Laws of Motion

Newton's Three Laws of Motion explain how forces create motion in sport. These laws are usually referred to as the Laws of Inertia, Acceleration, and Reaction.

- Law of Inertia: Newton's First Law of inertia states that objects tend to resist changes in their state of motion. An object in motion will tend to stay in motion and an object at rest will tend to stay at rest unless acted upon by a force. Example - The body of a player quickly sprinting down the field will tend to want to retain that motion unless muscular forces can overcome this inertia or a skater gliding on ice will continue gliding with the same speed and in the same direction, barring the action of an external force.

- Law of Acceleration: Newton's Second Law precisely explains how much motion a force creates. The acceleration (tendency of an object to change speed or direction) an object experiences is proportional to the size of the force and inversely proportional to the object's mass (F = ma). Example - When a ball is thrown, kicked, or struck with an implement, it tends to travel in the direction of the line of action of the applied force. Similarly, the greater the amount of force applied, the greater the speed the ball has. If a player improves leg strength through training while maintaining the same body mass, they will have an increased ability to accelerate the body using the legs, resulting in better agility and speed. This also relates to the ability to rotate segments.

- Law of Reaction: The Third Law states that for every action (force) there is an equal and opposite reaction force. This means that forces do not act alone, but occur in equal and opposite pairs between interacting bodies. Example - The force created by the legs "pushing" against the ground results in ground reaction forces in which the ground "pushes back" and allows the player to move across the court (As the Earth is much more massive than the player, the player accelerates and moves rapidly, while the Earth does not really accelerate or move at all). This action-reaction also occurs at impact with the ball as the force applied to the ball is matched with an equal and opposite force applied to the racket/body.

Momentum

Newton' Second Law is also related to the variable momentum, which is the product of an object's velocity and mass. Momentum is essentially the quantity of motion an object possesses. Momentum can be transferred from one object to another. There are different types of momentum which each have a different impact on the sport.

Linear Momentum

Linear momentum is momentum in a straight line e.g. linear momentum is created as the athlete sprints in a straight line down the 100m straight on the track.

Angular Momentum

Angular momentum is rotational momentum and is created by the rotations of the various body segments e.g. The open stance forehand uses significant angular momentum. The tremendous increase in the use of angular momentum in ground strokes and serves has had a significant impact on the game of tennis. One of the main reasons for the increase in power of the game today is the incorporation of angular momentum into ground stroke and serve techniques. In tennis, the angular momentum developed by the coordinated action of body segments transfers to the linear momentum of the racquet at impact.

Centre of Gravity

The Center of Gravity (COG) is an imaginary point around which body weight is evenly distributed. The center of gravity of the human body can change considerably because the segments of the body can move their masses with joint rotations. This concept is critical to understanding balance and stability and how gravity affects sport techniques.

The direction of the force of gravity through the body is downward, towards the center of the earth and through the COG. This line of gravity is important to understand and visualise when determining a person's ability to successfully maintain balance. When the line of gravity falls outside the Base of Support (BOS), then a reaction is needed in order to stay balanced.

The center of gravity of a squash racquet is a far simpler process and can usually be found by identifying the point where the racket balances on your finger or another narrow object.

Balance

Balance is the ability of a player to control their equilibrium or stability. You need to have a good understanding of both static and dynamic balance:

Static Balance

The ability to control the body while the body is stationary. It is the ability to maintain the body in some fixed posture. Static balance is the ability to maintain postural stability and orientation with center of mass over the base of support and body at rest.

Dynamic Balance

The ability to control the body during motion. Defining dynamic postural stability is more challenging, Dynamic balance is the ability to transfer the vertical projection of the center of gravity around the supporting base of support. Dynamic balance is the ability to maintain postural stability and orientation with center of mass over the base of support while the body parts are in motion.

Correct Biomechanics

Correct biomechanics provide efficient movement and may reduce the risk of injury. In sport, it is always good to consider abnormal or faulty biomechanics as a possible cause of injury. These abnormal biomechanics can be due to anatomical or functional abnormalities. Anatomical abnormalities such as leg length discrepancies cannot be changed, but the secondary effects can be addressed such as a shoe build up or orthotics for example. Functional abnormalities that can occur can be muscle imbalances after a long period of immobilisation.

In biomechanics the different planes of motion and axes are often referred to.

Incorrect technique can cause abnormal biomechanics which can lead to injuries. Below are some examples of the relationship between faulty technique and associated injuries:

Sport	Technique	Injury
Cricket	Mixed bowling action.	Pars interarticularis stress fractures.
Tennis	Excessive wrist action with backhand.	Extensor tendinopathy of the elbow.
Swimming	Decreased external rotation of the shoulder.	Rotator cuff tendinopathy.
Running	Anterior pelvic tilt.	Hamstring injuries.
Rowing	Change from bow side to stroke side.	Rib stress fractures.
Ballet	Poor turnout.	Hip Injuries.

Lower Limb Biomechanics

As humans, ambulation is our main form of movement, that is we walk upright and are very reliant on our legs to move us about. How the foot strikes the ground and the knock on effect this has up the lower limbs to the knee, hips, pelvis and low back in particular has become a subject of much debate and controversy in recent years.

Lower limb biomechanics refers to a complex interplay between the joints, muscles and nervous system which results in a certain patterning of movement, often referred to as 'alignment'. Much of the debate centers around what is considered 'normal' and what is considered 'abnormal' in biomechanical terms as well as the extent to which we should intervene should abnormal findings be found on assessment.

Foot and Ankle Biomechanics

The foot and ankle form a complex system which consists of 26 bones, 33 joints and more than 100 muscles, tendons and ligaments. It functions as a rigid structure for weight bearing and it can also function as a flexible structure to conform to uneven terrain. The foot and ankle provide various important functions which include: supporting body weight, providing balance, shock absorption, transferring ground reaction forces, compensating for proximal malalignment, and substituting hand function in individuals with upper extremity amputation/paralysis all which are key when involved with any exercise or sport involving the lower limbs.

Q Angle

An understanding of the normal anatomical and biomechanical features of the patellofemoral joint is essential to any evaluation of knee function. The Q angle formed by the vector for the combined pull of the quadriceps femoris muscle and the patellar tendon, is important because of the lateral pull it exerts on the patella.

The direction and magnitude of force produced by the quadriceps muscle have great influence on patellofemoral joint biomechanics. The line of force exerted by the quadriceps is lateral to the joint line mainly due to the large cross-sectional area and force potential of the vastus lateralis. Since there exists an association between patellofemoral pathology and excessive lateral tracking of the patella, assessing the overall lateral line of pull of the quadriceps relative to the patella is a meaningful clinical measure. Such a measure is referred to as the Quadriceps angle or Q angle.

Biomechanics of Gait

Sandra J. Shultz describes gait as: "someone's manner of ambulation or locomotion, involves the total body. Gait speed determines the contribution of each body segment. Normal walking speed primarily involves the lower extremities, with the arms and trunk providing stability and balance. The faster the speed, the more the body depends on the upper extremities and trunk for propulsion as well as balance and stability. The legs continue to do the most work as the joints produce greater ranges of motion through greater muscle responses. In the bipedal system the three major joints of the lower body and pelvis work with each other as muscles and momentum move the body forward. The degree to which the body's center of gravity moves during forward translation defines efficiency. The body's center moves both side to side and up and down during gait." Bipedal walking is an important characteristic of humans.

Upper Limb Biomechanics

Correct biomechanics are as important in upper limb activities as they are in lower limb activities. The capabilities of the upper extremity are varied and impressive. With the same basic anatomical structure of the arm, forearm, hand, and fingers, major league Baseball Pitchers pitch fastballs at 40 m/s, swimmers cross the English Channel, gymnasts perform the iron cross, and olympic boxers in weight classes ranging from flyweight to super heavyweight showed a range of 447 to 1,066 pounds of peak punching force.

The structure of the upper extremity is composed of the shoulder girdle and the upper limb. The shoulder girdle consists of the scapula and clavicle, and the upper limb is composed of the arm, forearm, wrist, hand, and fingers. However, a kinematic chain extends from the cervical and upper thoracic spine to the fingertips. Only when certain multiple segments are completely fixed can these parts possibly function independently in mechanical roles.

Scapulohumeral Rhythm

Scapulohumeral rhythm (also referred to as glenohumeral rhythm) is the kinematic interaction between the scapula and the humerus, first published by Codman in the 1930's. This interaction is important for the optimal function of the shoulder. When there is a change of the normal position of the scapula relative to the humerus, this can cause a dysfunction of the scapulohumeral rhythm. The change of the normal position is also called scapular dyskinesia. Various studies of the mechanism of the shoulder joint that have attempted to describe the global motion capacity of the shoulder refer to that description.

Sport Specific Biomechanics

Running Biomechanics

Running is similar to walking in terms of locomotive activity. However, there are key differences. Having the ability to walk does not mean that the individual has the ability to run. There are some differences between the gait and run cycle - the gait cycle is one third longer in time, the ground reaction force is smaller in the gait cycle (so the load is lower), and the velocity is much higher. In running, there is also just one stance phase while in stepping there are two. Shock absorption is also much larger in comparison to walking. This explains why runners have more overload injuries.

Running requires:

- Greater balance.

- Greater muscle strength.

- Greater joint range of movement.

Cycling Biomechanics

Cycling was initially invented by Baron Carl von Drais in 1817, but not as we know it. This was a machine which initially had two wheels that were connected by a wooden plank with a rudder device for steering. It involved people running along the ground whilst sitting down; giving them the name of a 'running machine' (in all senses) or a velocipede. This was solely used by the male population at the time of invention. The velocipede then made a huge design development in the 1860s at the Michaux factory in Paris. They added leaver arms to the front wheel which were propelled by pedals at the feet. This was the first conventional bicycle, and since then and up until the current day the bicycle has made great design and technological advances. A survey in 2014 estimated that over 43% of the United Kingdom population have or have access to a bike and 8% of the population aged 5 and above cycled 3 or more times a week. With such a large amount of people cycling, whether it be professional, recreational or for commuting this increase the chance of developing an injury, so it is time we understood the biomechanics of cycling.

Baseball Pitching Biomechanics

Baseball pitching is one of the most intensely studying athletic motions. Although the focus has been more on the shoulder movement, entire body movement is required to perform baseball pitching. Throwing is also considered one of the fastest human motions performed, and maximum humeral internal rotation velocity reaches about 7000 to 75000/second.

Tennis Biomechanics

Tennis biomechanics is a very complex task. Consider hitting a tennis ball. First, the athlete needs to see the ball coming off their opponent's racket. Then, in order, they have to judge the speed, spin, trajectory and, most importantly, the direction of the tennis ball. The player then needs to adjust their body position quickly to move around the ball. As the player prepares to hit the ball the body is in motion, the ball is moving both in a linear and rotation direction if there is spin on the ball, and the racquet is also in motion. The player must coordinate all these movements in approximately a half a second so they strike the ball as close to the center of the racket in order to produce the desired spin, speed and direction for return of the ball. A mistake in any of these movements can create an error.

COMPUTATIONAL BIOMECHANICS

Computational biomechanics is a promising research field, which provides thorough treatment from foot, ankle, knee, hip, lower limb, spine, to head and teeth, as well as bone and muscle at the tissue level. It informs about complex biomechanical behaviors of normal and pathological human joints to surface new methods of orthopedictreatment and rehabilitation. It provides novel link between surgeons and machines, which enables them to map and carry out surgical interventions with more accuracy and lesser amount of trauma. Computer-integrated surgery systems could help to improve clinical outcomes and the efficient healthcare delivery. It also helps in getting footing for computer-integrated medicine by extracting clinically important information regarding the physical status of the underlying biology at cell, tissue, organ, and organism level and integrating information with molecules of body.

BIOFLUID DYNAMICS

Biofluid dynamics may be considered as the discipline of biological engineering or biomedical engineering in which the fundamental principles of fluid dynamics are used to explain the mechanisms of biological flows and their interrelationships with physiological processes, in health and in diseases/disorder. It can be considered as the conjuncture of mechanical engineering and biological engineering. It spans from cells to organs, covering diverse aspects of the functionality of systemic physiology, including cardiovascular, respiratory, reproductive, urinary, musculoskeletal and neurological systems etc.

Biofluid dynamics and its simulations in computational fluid dynamics (CFD) apply to both internal as well as external flows. Internal flows such as cardiovascular blood flow and respiratory airflow, and external flows such as flying and aquatic locomotion (i.e., swimming). Biological fluid Dynamics (or Biofluid Dynamics) involves the study of the motion of biological fluids (e.g. blood flow in arteries, animal flight, fish swimming, etc.). It can be either circulatory system or respiratory systems. Understanding the circulatory system is one of the major areas of research. The respiratory system is very closely linked to the circulatory system and is very complex to study and understand. The study of Biofluid Dynamics is also directed towards finding solutions to some of the human body related diseases and disorders. The usefulness of the subject can also be understood by seeing the use of Biofluid Dynamics in the areas of physiology in order to explain how living things work and about their motions, in developing an understanding of the origins and development of various diseases related to human body and diagnosing them, in finding the cure for the diseases related to cardiovascular and pulmonary systems.

Basic Principles of Fluid Dynamics

A fluid is defined as a substance that deforms continuously under application of a shearing stress, regardless of how small the stress is. Blood is a primary example of a biological fluid. Air can also be considered as biological fluid as it flows in lungs and the synovial fluid between the knee joints is also an example of a biological fluid. Types of Fluids Fluids can be classified into four basic types. They are:

- Ideal Fluid.

- Real Fluid.

- Newtonian Fluid.

- Non-Newtonian fluid.

An Ideal Fluid is a fluid that has no viscosity, means it will offer no resistance, pragmatically this type of fluid does not exist. It is incompressible in nature. Real fluids are compressible in nature. They offer some resistance and thus have viscosity. All Fluids existing are real fluids. A Newtonian Fluid is a fluid whose viscous shear stresses (acting between different layers of fluid and between the fluid layer and surface over which it is flowing) are directly proportional to the rate of change of velocity of the flow of the fluid with respect to the distance in the transverse direction (distance measured perpendicular to the flow), also known as velocity gradient. The constant of proportionality is known as the dynamic viscosity of the fluid denoted by 'μ'. The functional relationship between viscous shear stress and velocity gradient is linear in a Newtonian fluid. This relationship may be written as:

$$\tau = -\mu \frac{du}{dy}$$

Where τ = viscous shear stress

μ = dynamic viscosity of the fluid

$\dfrac{du}{dy}$ = velocity gradient across the flow

A Non-Newtonian fluid is a fluid which is different from the Newtonian fluid as the viscosity of non-Newtonian fluids is dependent on shear rate or shear rate history. In a non-Newtonian fluid, the relation between the shear stress and the shear rate is different and can even be time-dependent (Time Dependent Viscosity). Therefore, a constant coefficient of viscosity cannot be defined.

Non-Newtonian fluids change their viscosity or flow behavior under stress. If a force is applied to such fluids, the sudden application of stress can cause them to get thicker and act like a solid, or in some cases, it results in the opposite behavior and they may get runnier than they were before. Removal of the stress causes them to return to their earlier state. Not all non-Newtonian Fluids behave in the same way when stress is applied – some become more solid, others more fluid. Some non-Newtonian fluids react as a result of the amount of stress applied, while others react as a result of the length of time that stress is applied. The generalized power law for all fluids can be written as:

$$\tau = K \left(\frac{dy}{dx} \right)^n$$

Where K = flow consistency index

n = Fluid behavior index, n=1 for Newtonian fluids

- Thixotropic Fluid: Its viscosity decreases with stress over time. Example - Honey – keep stirring, and solid honey becomes liquid.

- Rheopectic Fluid: Its viscosity increases with stress over time. Example - Cream – the longer it is whipped, the thicker it gets.

- Shear Thinning Fluid: Its viscosity decreases with increased stress. Example – Blood, Tomato sauce.

- Dilatant or shear thickening Fluid: Its viscosity increases with increased stress. Example – Oobleck (a mixture of cornstarch and water), Quicksand.

A Bingham plastic is neither a fluid nor a solid. A Bingham plastic can withstand a finite shear load and flow like a fluid when that shear stress is exceeded. Toothpaste and mayonnaise are examples of Bingham plastics. Blood is also a Bingham plastic and behaves as a solid at shear rates very close to zero. The yield stress for blood is very small, approximately in the range from 0.005 to 0.01 N/m2.

Reynolds number of the flow is defined as the ratio of inertia forces to viscous forces. Mathematically it is written as:

$$Re = \frac{\rho v d}{\mu}$$

Where,

ρ = density of fluid.

v = velocity of fluid.

d = characteristic length.

μ = dynamic viscosity of fluid.

The Reynolds number helps us to predict the transition between laminar and turbulent flows. Laminar flow is highly organized flow along streamlines. As velocity increases, flow can become disorganized and chaotic. This is known as turbulent flow. Laminar flow occurs in flow environments where Re < 2000. Turbulent flow is present in circumstances under which Re > 4000. The range of 2000 < Re < 4000 is known as the transition range. Most blood flow in humans is laminar, having a Re of 300 or less, it is possible for turbulence to occur at very high flow rates in the descending aorta, for example, in highly conditioned athletes. Turbulence is also common in pathological conditions such as heart murmurs and stenotic heart valves. Stenotic means narrowed, and a stenotic heart valve is one in which the narrowing of the valve is a result of the plaque formation on the valve.

The Womersley number, or alpha parameter, is another dimensionless parameter like the Prandtl number or Reynolds number that has been used in the study of fluid dynamics. This parameter represents a ratio of transient to viscous forces, just as the Reynolds number represented a ratio of inertial to viscous forces. A characteristic frequency represents the time dependence of the parameter. The Womersley number may be written as:

$$\alpha = r\sqrt{\frac{\omega}{\vartheta}}$$

Where,

α = Womersely Number.

r = vessel radius.

ω = fundamental frequency.

ϑ = kinematic viscosity.

The flow profile becomes blunter near the centerline of the vessel in high frequency flows, because the inertia forces become more important than viscous forces. But viscous forces are still important near the wall as here the velocity of the flow is almost zero due to the effect of the wall and the no-slip condition. Moreover, it can be shown that the transient forces become relatively more important than viscous forces as the animal size increases.

The Cardiovascular System

The Heart, arteries, and veins (a network of tubes to carry blood) constitute the cardio-vascular system or circulatory system of our body which transports the blood through-out the body. The heart can be thought of as a muscular pump, consisting of four chambers, and pulsatile muscles which pump and circulates the blood through the vas-culature. Arteries, arterioles, capillaries, venules, and veins make up the vasculature. The cardiovascular system circulates about 5 liters of blood at a rate of approximately 6 l/m. The pulmonary and the systemic circulations are the two parts of the vascula-ture. The pulmonary circulation system consists of the network of blood vessels from the right heart to the lungs and back to the left heart. The rest of the blood flow loop is called systemic circulation system. The pulmonary and systemic circulations take the blood through large arteries first and then branches into smaller arteries before reaching arterioles and capillaries. After capillaries, the blood enters the venules before joining smaller veins first and then larger veins before reaching the right heart. Thus completing the cycle of blood going to heart and then coming from it and going to all parts of the body. The tricuspid valve, right heart (right ventricle), pulmonary valve, pulmonary artery, lungs, pulmonary veins and right heart are the elements of the Pul-monary Circulation System. The process of gas exchange, that is, exchange of carbon dioxide with oxygen in the lungs is the main function of the pulmonary system. The de-oxygenated blood from the right ventricle is pumped to the lungs where the capil-laries surrounding the alveole sacks exchange carbon dioxide for oxygen. The red blood cells and the hemoglobin present in the blood, which is the main carrier of oxygen in the blood are responsible for this exchange of gases before they are carried to the left ventricle of the heart. The systemic circulation is responsible for taking the oxygenated blood to various organs and tissues via the arterial tree before taking the deoxygenated blood to the right ventricle using the venous system (a network of veins). Arteries carry the oxygenated blood while the veins carry the deoxygenated blood.

Elements of Blood and Blood Rheology

The fluids associated with the human body include air, oxygen, carbon dioxide, water, solvents, solutions, suspensions, serum, lymph, and blood. The major body fluid which acts as the lifeline of the living organisms is "Blood". Blood is an extremely complex bi-ological fluid. It consists of blood cells suspended in plasma and other different types of cells which include white blood cells, platelets etc. The blood flow in arteries and veins are closely linked to the blood vessel properties. Carrying the oxygen and nutrients to vari-ous tissues and organs of our body, delivering carbon dioxide to the lungs and accepting oxygen, bringing the metabolic by products to the kidneys, regulating the body's defence mechanism, that is, the immune system and facilitating an effective heat and mass transfer across the body are some of the major functions which blood performs in the human body. Blood consists of the red blood cells or erythrocytes, white blood cells or leukocytes, and platelets or thrombocytes. The cells which are involved primarily in the transport of oxygen and carbon dioxide are known as Erythrocytes. The cells which are involved primarily in phagocytosis (the process of destruction of unknown particulate matter) and immune responses are known as Leukocytes; thrombocytes are the components of blood which are involved in blood clotting. In addition to these 55 to 60 percent of blood by volume consists of plasma. Plasma is the transparent, amber-colored liquid in which the cellular components of blood are suspended. Plasma contains constituents such as proteins, electrolytes, hormones, and nutrients. The serum is blood plasma from which clotting factors have been removed. Blood accounts for 6 to 8 percent of body weight in normal, healthy humans. The density of blood is slightly greater than the density of water at approximately 1060 kg/m3. The increased density comes from the increased density of a red blood cell compared with the density of water or plasma. Rheology is the study of the deformation and flow of matter. Blood Rheology is the study of blood, especially the properties associated with the deformation and flow of blood. Blood is a non-Newtonian fluid. However, often the non-Newtonian effect is very small due to various reasons. Thus, it is important to know about the blood rheology. One of the characteristics of blood that affects the work required to cause the blood to flow through the arteries is the viscosity of blood. The viscosity of blood is in the range of 3 to 6 cP, or 0.003 to 0.006 Ns/m2. Blood is a non-Newtonian fluid, which means that the viscosity of blood is not a constant with respect to the rate of shearing strain. In addition to the rate of shearing strain, the viscosity of blood is also dependent on temperature and on the volume percentage of blood that consists of red blood cells. If blood is made stationary for several seconds then clotting begins in the blood, as a result of which the viscosity of the blood increases. When the stationary state is disturbed with increasing shear rate, the clot formation is destroyed and the viscosity decreases. Moreover, the orientation of red blood cells present in the blood also affects the viscosity of blood. Thus, we can say that blood is a shear thinning fluid, i.e., viscosity decreases with increase in shear rate. Beyond a shear rate of about $100s^{-1}$, the viscosity is nearly constant and the blood behaves like a Newtonian fluid. Blood is a viscoelastic material, i.e., viscous and elastic because the effective viscosity of blood not only depends on the shear rate but also on the history of shear rate. It is also important to note that the normal blood flows much more easily compared to rigid particles, for the same particle volume fraction. This is due to the fact that red blood cells can accommodate by deforming in order to pass by one another.

Fåhræus-Lindqvist Effect

Robert (Robin) Sanno Fåhræus, a Swedish pathologist, and hematologist, and Johan Torsten Lindqvist, a Swedish physician, observed that when blood flows through vessels smaller than about 1.5 mm in diameter, the apparent viscosity of the fluid decreases. The viscosity of blood decreases as the percent of the diameter of a vessel occupied by the cell-free layer increases. However, when the diameter of the tube approaches the diameter of the erythrocyte, the viscosity increases dramatically. For blood flow through tubes less than approximately 1 mm in diameter, the viscosity is not constant with respect to the tube diameter. Therefore, blood behaves as a non-Newtonian fluid in such blood vessels.

Applications of Biofluid Dynamics

Biofluid Dynamics refers to the study of fluid Dynamics of basic biological fluids such as blood, air etc. and has immense applications in the field of diagnosing, treating and certain surgical procedures related to the disorders/diseases which originate in the body relating to cardiovascular, pulmonary, synovial systems etc. The different types of cardiovascular diseases include Aneurysms, Angina, Atherosclerosis, Stroke, Different types of Cerebrovascular disease, Heart Failure, Coronary Heart diseases and Myo-cardial infarction or Heart attacks. The Computational Fluid dynamics (CFD) models prepared through software, of the arteries, veins etc. not only lead to the identifica-tion of properties of flowing blood inside arteries but also changes in viscosity can be identified which may be the result of certain underlying disease/disorder. Moreover, the stress concentration and the distribution of stresses in different biological systems carrying fluids can also be identified. This has led to a greater degree of assistance to biomedical engineers in recognizing the cause of certain diseases and thus they can eas-ily search for the method of cure for that disease/disorder. Also, this has led to a greater degree of good research in the fields of biotechnology, Bio-Mechanics etc.

NANOBIOMECHANICS

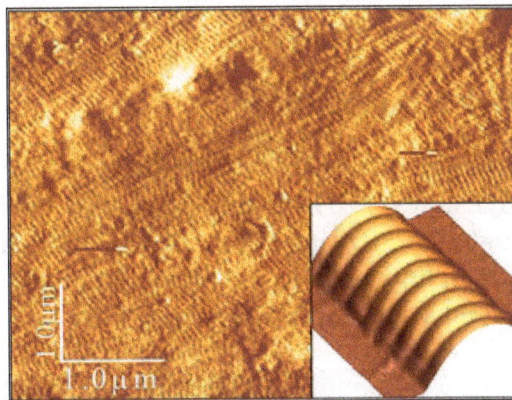

High resolution AFM image of cortical bone and single collagen fibril (inset).

Nanobiomechanics (also bionanomechanics) is an emerging field in nanoscience and biomechanics that combines the powerful tools of nanomechanics to explore funda-mental science of biomaterials and biomechanics.

Since the introduction by its founder Yuan-Cheng Fung, the field of biomechanics has become one of the branches of mechanics and bioscience. For many years, biomechanics has examined tissue. Through advancements in nanoscience, the scale of the forces that could be measured and also the scale of observation of biomaterials was reduced to "nano" and "pico" level. Consequently, it became possible to measure the mechanical properties of biological materials at nanoscale.

Most of the biological materials have different hierarchical levels, and the smallest ones refer to the nanoscale. For example, bone has up to seven levels of biological organization, and the smallest level, i.e., single collagen fibril and hydroxylapatite minerals have dimensions well below 100 nm. Therefore, being able to probe properties at this small scales provides a great opportunity for better understanding the fundamental properties of these materials. For example, measurements have shown that nanomechanical heterogeneity exists even within single collagen fibrils as small as 100 nm.

One of the other most relevant topics in this field is measurement of tiny forces on living cells to recognize changes caused by different diseases. For example, it has been shown that red blood cells infected by malaria are 10 times stiffer than normal cells. Likewise, it has been shown that cancer cells are 70 percent softer than normal cells. Early signs of aging cartilage and osteoarthritis has been shown by looking at the changes in the tissue at the nanoscale.

Methods and Instrumentation

The common methods in nanobiomechanics are atomic force microscope, optical tweezers, and magnetic twisting cytometry.

Examples of relevant materials are bone and its hierarchical constituents such as single collagen fibrils, single living cells, actin filaments and microtubules, and synthetic peptide nanotubes.

Computational Nanobiomechanics

In addition to experimental aspect, research has been expanding through computational methods. Molecular dynamics (MD) simulations have provided a wealth of knowledge in this area. Although, the MD simulation are still limited to a small number of atoms and molecules, due to limitation in the computational performance, they have proved to be an instrumental branch of this emerging field.

NEURO BIOMECHANICS

Neuro Biomechanics is based upon the research of bioengineering researchers, neuro-surgery, orthopedic surgery and biomechanists. Neuro Biomechanics are utilized by neurosurgeons, orthopedic surgeons and primarily by integrated physical medicine practitioners. Practitioners are focused on aiding people in the restoration of biomechanics of the skeletal system in order to measurably improve nervous system function, health, function, quality of life, reduce pain and the progression of degenerative joint and disc disease.

Neuro: of or having to do with the nervous system. Nervous System: An organ system that coordinates the activities of muscles, monitors organs, constructs and processes data received from the senses and initiates actions. The human nervous system coordinates the functions of itself and all organ systems including but not limited to the cardiovascular system, respiratory system, skin, digestive system, immune system, hormonal, metabolic, musculoskeletal, endocrine system, blood and reproductive system. Optimal function of the organism as a whole depends upon the proper function of the nervous system.

Biomechanics: (biology, physics) The branch of biophysics that deals with the mechanics of the human or animal body; especially concerned with muscles and the skeleton. The study of biomechanical influences upon nervous system function and load bearing joints.

BIOMECHATRONICS

Biomechatronics is an applied interdisciplinary science that aims to integrate biology, mechanics, and electronics. It also encompasses the fields of robotics and neuroscience. Biomechatronic devices encompass a wide range of applications from the development of prosthetic limbs to engineering solutions concerning respiration, vision, and the cardiovascular system.

Biomechatronics mimics how the human body works. For example, four different steps must occur to be able to lift the foot to walk. First, impulses from the motor center of the brain are sent to the foot and leg muscles. Next the nerve cells in the feet send information, providing feedback to the brain, enabling it to adjust the muscle groups or amount of force required to walk across the ground. Different amounts of force are applied depending on the type of surface being walked across. The leg's muscle spindle nerve cells then sense and send the position of the floor back up to the brain. Finally, when the foot is raised to step, signals are sent to muscles in the leg and foot to set it down.

Biosensors

Biosensors are used to detect what the user wants to do or their intentions and motions. In some devices the information can be relayed by the user's nervous system or muscle system. This information is related by the biosensor to a controller which can be located inside or outside the biomechatronic device. In addition biosensors receive information about the limb position and force from the limb and actuator. Biosensors come in a variety of forms. They can be wires which detect electrical activity, needle electrodes implanted in muscles, and electrode arrays with nerves growing through them.

Mechanical Sensors

The purpose of the mechanical sensors is to measure information about the biomechatronic device and relate that information to the biosensor or controller.

Controller

The controller in a biomechatronic device relays the user's intentions to the actuators. It also interprets feedback information to the user that comes from the biosensors and mechanical sensors. The other function of the controller is to control the biomechatronic device's movements.

Actuator

The actuator is an artificial muscle. Its job is to produce force and movement. Depending on whether the device is orthotic or prosthetic the actuator can be a motor that assists or replaces the user's original muscle.

Research

Biomechatronics is a rapidly growing field but as of now there are very few labs which conduct research. The Shirley Ryan AbilityLab (formerly the Rehabilitation Institute of Chicago), University of California at Berkeley, MIT, Stanford University, and University of Twente in the Netherlands are the researching leaders in biomechatronics. Three main areas are emphasized in the current research.

- Analyzing human motions, which are complex, to aid in the design of biomechatronic devices.
- Studying how electronic devices can be interfaced with the nervous system.
- Testing the ways to use living muscle tissue as actuators for electronic devices.

Analyzing Motions

A great deal of analysis over human motion is needed because human movement is very complex. MIT and the University of Twente are both working to analyze these movements. They are doing this through a combination of computer models, camera systems, and electromyograms.

Interfacing

Interfacing allows biomechatronics devices to connect with the muscle systems and nerves of the user in order send and receive information from the device. This is a technology that is not available in ordinary orthotics and prosthetics devices. Groups at the University of Twente and University of Malaya are making drastic steps in this department. Scientists there have developed a device which will help to treat paralysis and stroke victims who are unable to control their foot while walking. The researchers are also nearing a breakthrough which would allow a person with an amputated leg to control their prosthetic leg through their stump muscles.

BIOTRIBOLOGY

Biotribology is the science of tribology applied to functioning biological systems, in particular, the synovial joints and their artificial replacements. Tribology is defined as the science and technology of interacting surfaces in relative motion, and comprises three related areas: friction, wear and lubrication.

Understanding the wear mechanism is important in design of appropriate strategies to reduce wear debris and associated problems, like aseptic loosening. A wide range of laboratory equipment, test methods and measuring systems have been developed for study of the wear mechanisms in total hip replacement. For example, screening analysis, where pin-on-disc and pin-on-plate machines are used to assess the wear behaviour of new combinations of materials at an early phase; and joint simulation, using equipment that simulates the functioning of a human joint.

Pin-on-disc machines are widely used in tribology to evaluate the nature of wear and friction of material pairs under well-controlled steady-state conditions of load, sliding speed and environment. Pin-on-plate machines sacrifice the steady sliding speed between specimens, but partially simulate the reciprocating action broadly associated with the hip joint.

Joint simulators reproduce the three-dimensional loading and motion patterns experienced by hip joints and provide a lubricant environment similar to synovial fluid. This kind of equipment allows a comparative performance evaluation of hip joints of different designs and material combinations.

Friction

Friction is generally explained as the resistance to relative motion between articulating surfaces. It is the main cause of wear and energy loss. An energy input is provided for the motion of sliding surfaces and maintaining the motion. This energy is dissipated into the system, mainly as frictional heat that causes property changes in sliding materials, tissue damage, and changes in lubricant properties such as protein precipitation especially in the biotribological zone.

A deep understanding of friction and wear processes first requires the investigation of the influence of numerous effects accompanying the friction process, i.e., mechanical, electrical, hydroacoustic, physicochemical, and other effects, and their influence on physicochemical properties, structure of working surfaces, etc. Friction is generally classified as static friction, sliding friction, and rolling friction.

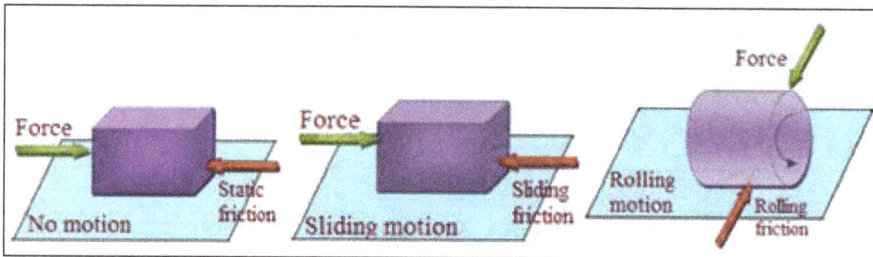

Scheme of friction force and motion.

In static friction, there is no motion. To slide a contacting body over another, a tangential force must be overcome which is named as friction force(F). It acts on the sliding surface plane and is usually proportional to the normal force (N):

$$F = \mu \cdot N$$

The proportionality constant termed as the coefficient of friction (μ) is used for quantifying sliding or kinetic friction, and it is defined as the ratio between the friction force F and the normal load N:

$$\mu = \frac{F}{N}$$

The coefficient of friction generally ranges from 0.03 for well-lubricated bearing to 1 for dry sliding. These values change according to operating parameters, such as sliding speed, applied load or contact pressure, temperature, presence of lubricant, and the properties of materials in contact such as surface roughness of sliding pairs.

For comfortable walking, the coefficient of friction must be 0.2–0.3; on ice walking, the μ-value between shoe and ice pair nearly becomes 0.05. In a synovial joint, with the very efficient natural lubrication, the coefficient of friction is 0.02.

Surfaces are not perfect at the microscopic level. Peaks, valleys, asperities, and depressions can be seen at high magnification even on the best polished surface. When these two surfaces are brought together, they touch from the tips of the surface asperities. At that point, adhesion or cold welding, which generally refers to resistance to separating bodies from each other, may occur, and plastic deformation may take place on a very local scale.

To start the sliding motion, these formations must be broken by the friction force. The main contribution to friction action is extended by adhesion and deformation, but additional contributions may occur, such as wear debris, presence of oxides, or adsorbed films.

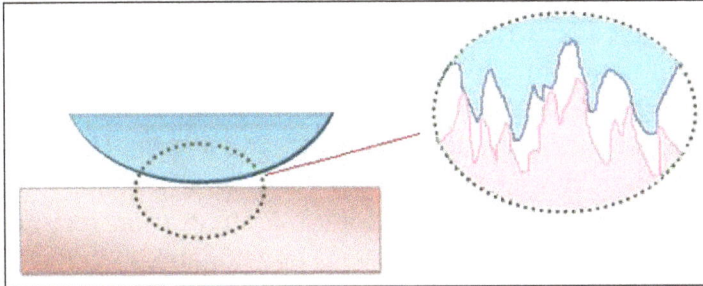

Microscopic detail of a real surface contact.

Lubrication

The main purpose of using lubricant is reducing the effect of normal and shear stresses on the solid surface contact. Lubrication is one of the most effective ways of minimizing friction and delaying wear. Unfortunately, it is not the exact solution of the wear because wear occurs even with lubrication. Especially abrasive wear and delamination problem may occur under lubricated conditions.

Different types of lubrication regimes may arise between the sliding surfaces. In all lubricating modes, the surfaces are separated by a solid, a semisolid, a pressurized liquid, or the gaseous form of a lubricating film. Dry-film (solid-film) lubrication is a system in which a coating of solid-state lubricant separates the sliding surfaces and the lubricant itself wears away. Boundary lubrication is the regime in which the interacting surfaces react with the lubricant components. Each surface is covered by a chemically bonded fluid or a semisolid film that may or may not separate opposing surfaces. In thin-film lubrication, the lubricant usually is not bonded to the surfaces and it does not separate sliding surfaces. Moreover, lubricant viscosity affects friction and wear. In fluid-film lubrication, the sliding surfaces are separated by a fluid film and the physical properties of the lubricant such as viscosity and pressure viscosity designate the performance of the lubricated surfaces. This lubrication regime can be divided into two subcategories such as hydrodynamic lubrication and elastohydrodynamic lubrication. Hydrodynamic lubrication is a regime in which the formation of the fluid film depends on the shape and relative motion of the sliding surfaces with sufficient pressure for separating the surfaces. For the mathematical explanation of hydrodynamic lubrication, an equation derived by Reynolds known as the "Reynolds equation" is used. In elastohydrodynamic lubrication, friction and film thickness between the sliding surfaces are defined by the elastic properties of the contacting bodies. Although fluid-film lubrication is a desired regime, the boundary lubrication cannot be avoided. Boundary lubrication occurs during starting up and stopping stages of the motion. In mixed lubrication, boundary and the fluid film lubricated regions are considered simultaneously.

To minimize the friction and wear of the sliding surfaces, understanding and determining lubrication mechanism are very important tools for the optimization of the bearing materials and geometries, both in engineering system and artificial joints. For the theoretical prediction of the lubrication regime, some classical engineering methods can be applied to artificial joints. At that point, it is necessary to provide some basic information about geometrical and surface features of hip joint. Joints in a human body may be classified anatomically and physiologically such as plane, ball-in-socket, ellipsoid, hinge, condylar, pivot, and saddle. Hip joint is considered as ball-in-socket geometry where contacting surfaces fit together. In theoretical calculations sometimes ball-on-plane equivalent configuration may be used for simplifying the geometry. In ball-in-socket types of geometries, contacting bodies have same diameters but with a clearance between the elements for suitable fit of the bodies and tribological reasons. R_{head}, R_{cup}, and $c = R_{cup} - R_{head}$ represent the femoral head radii, acetabular cup radii, and radial clearance, respectively. Another important parameter of sliding bodies is the average surface roughness R_a of the frictional surfaces. It is relevant for the determination of the lubrication regime, Schematic drawing of relation between the surface roughness and the film thickness can be seen in Figure.

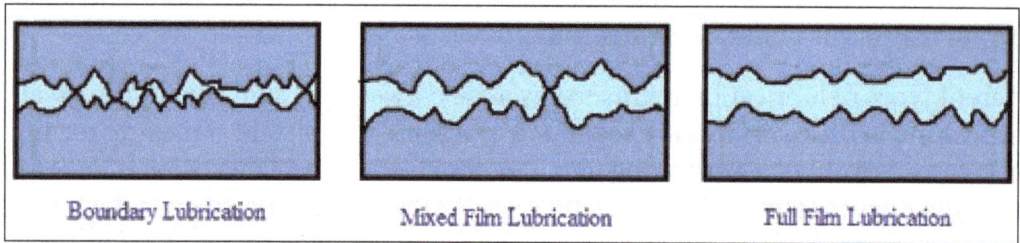

| Boundary Lubrication | Mixed Film Lubrication | Full Film Lubrication |

Schematic drawing of relation between the surface roughness and the film thickness.

The parameter λ, which is the ratio between the minimum film thickness h_{min} and the composite roughness of the sliding surfaces R_a, is generally used for determining the distance between the sliding surface asperities:

$$\lambda = \frac{h_{min}}{R_a} = \frac{h_{min}}{\left[(R_{a\,head})^2 + (R_{a\,cup})^2\right]^{1/2}}$$

With the evaluation of λ, the lubrication regime can be identified in the following ranges:

- $0.1 < \lambda < 1$: boundary lubrication.

- $1 \leq \lambda \leq 3$: mixed lubrication.

- $\lambda > 3$: full film lubrication.

The precision measurement of surface roughness for both femoral head and acetabular cup is important for the accurate determination of λ.

For the determination of film thickness, the following equation formulated for engineering can be used:

$$\frac{h_{min}}{R'} = 2.8\left(\frac{\eta u}{E'R'}\right)^{0.65}\left(\frac{W}{E'R'^2}\right)^{-0.21}$$

where R' is the equivalent radius that depends on the femoral head radius R_{head} and the radial clearance c.

$$\frac{1}{R'} = \frac{1}{R_{head}} - \frac{1}{R_{cup}} = \frac{c}{R_{head}(R_{head}+c)}$$

In the ball-on-plane equivalent configuration, the entraining velocity (u) can be calculated from the angular velocity of the femoral head (ω):

$$u = \frac{\omega R_{head}}{2}$$

The equivalent elastic modulus (E') can be determined by following equation:

$$\frac{1}{E'} = \left(\frac{1}{2}\frac{1-v^2_{head}}{E_{head}} + \frac{1-v^2_{cup}}{E_{cup}}\right)$$

where E_{head}, v_{head} and E_{cup}, v_{cup} are the Young's modulus and Poisson ratio of the femoral head and acetabular cup material, respectively.

For the prediction of lubrication between the femoral head and acetabular cup bearing surfaces and its effect on friction, generated during articulation, the Stribeck diagram can be used. In this diagram, the relation between the lubrication and friction is commonly illustrated:

$$z = \frac{\eta u r}{W}$$

where z is the Sommerfeld number, η is the lubricant viscosity, u is the sliding speed, r is the radius, and W is the load.

Traditionally, the Stribeck curve is divided into three regions. Boundary lubrication is seen when the thickness of the lubricating film is less than or equal to the average surface roughness of the articulating surfaces. When the thickness of the lubrication film increases, a transition stage, called mixed lubrication, is generated. The articulating surfaces are separated from each other while in contact with some asperities, and the combination of the fluid film and boundary lubrication can be seen in this regime. Full fluid film lubrication occurs with the continuous decrease in the friction coefficient, and the articulating surfaces are completely separated.

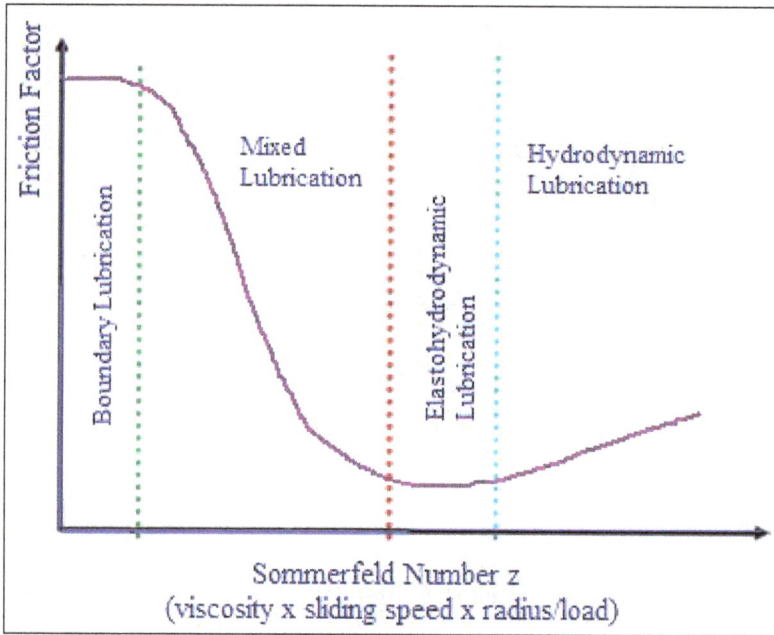

The Stribeck curve.

Wear

Wear is defined as the progressive loss of material from the surface of a body. It is a complex phenomenon that involves multifarious events in a wildly unpredictable manner. Numerous types of wear have already been defined in different studies related to tribology. Although it is difficult to classify wear types without considering mating materials, for a general classification wear can be divided into five different groups, such as abrasive, adhesive, surface fatigue, erosive, and corrosive.

Abrasive wear is generally categorized according to contact types of the surfaces such as two-body and three-body wear. When the asperities of the harder surface abrade the softer one, it is called as two-body abrasion. If there are hard particles trapped between surfaces and abrade one or both of the surfaces, it is known as three-body abrasion. Adhesive wear occurs due to high local friction that leads to tearing and fracture. This type of wear is generally defined as transfer of material from one surface to another during relative motion. The particles, broken away from one surface, may attach to another surface and act as an abrasive. This kind of wear may be seen between ceramic, polymers, and metallic material pairs or their combinations. Corrosive wear is the wear that contains both mechanical wear and chemical reaction in which metal ions are released. Besides the chemical and electrochemical reactions, environmental conditions govern the oxidative wear. Fatigue wear is the displacement of the particles from the microscopic contact area of material surface by cyclic loading. It may lead to the generation of debris from the surface or cracks' propagation into the bulk material. Erosive wear is the loss of surface layer of the material caused by hard particles attacking to the surface. The attacking particles may be in solid, liquid, or slurry form. This type of wear may involve plastic deformation and brittle fracture. Erosive wear is similar to abrasive wear and generally be confused with it, but there is a definite distinction between erosive and abrasive wear. In erosive wear, the force is transferred to the surface by the particles due to their slowing down, while in abrasive wear, the force is externally applied. This kind of wear is not common in hip joints.

References

- Biomechanics-In-Sport: physio-pedia.com, Retrieved 19 June, 2019

- Computational-biomechanics: sciencedirect.com, Retrieved 16 May, 2019

- Minary-Jolandan, Majid; Yu, Min-Feng (2009). "Nanomechanical heterogeneity in the gap and overlap regions of type I collagen fibrils with implications for bone heterogeneity". Biomacromolecules. 10 (9): 2565–70. doi:10.1021/bm900519v. PMID 19694448

- Brooker, Graham (2012). Introduction to Biomechatronics. University of Sydney, Australia. ISBN 978-1-891121-27-2

- Biotribology, materials-science: sciencedirect.com, Retrieved 05 April, 2019

- Biotribology-of-artificial-hip-joints, advances-in-tribology: intechopen.com, Retrieved 28 August, 2019

Permissions

All chapters in this book are published with permission under the Creative Commons Attribution Share Alike License or equivalent. Every chapter published in this book has been scrutinized by our experts. Their significance has been extensively debated. The topics covered herein carry significant information for a comprehensive understanding. They may even be implemented as practical applications or may be referred to as a beginning point for further studies.

We would like to thank the editorial team for lending their expertise to make the book truly unique. They have played a crucial role in the development of this book. Without their invaluable contributions this book wouldn't have been possible. They have made vital efforts to compile up to date information on the varied aspects of this subject to make this book a valuable addition to the collection of many professionals and students.

This book was conceptualized with the vision of imparting up-to-date and integrated information in this field. To ensure the same, a matchless editorial board was set up. Every individual on the board went through rigorous rounds of assessment to prove their worth. After which they invested a large part of their time researching and compiling the most relevant data for our readers.

The editorial board has been involved in producing this book since its inception. They have spent rigorous hours researching and exploring the diverse topics which have resulted in the successful publishing of this book. They have passed on their knowledge of decades through this book. To expedite this challenging task, the publisher supported the team at every step. A small team of assistant editors was also appointed to further simplify the editing procedure and attain best results for the readers.

Apart from the editorial board, the designing team has also invested a significant amount of their time in understanding the subject and creating the most relevant covers. They scrutinized every image to scout for the most suitable representation of the subject and create an appropriate cover for the book.

The publishing team has been an ardent support to the editorial, designing and production team. Their endless efforts to recruit the best for this project, has resulted in the accomplishment of this book. They are a veteran in the field of academics and their pool of knowledge is as vast as their experience in printing. Their expertise and guidance has proved useful at every step. Their uncompromising quality standards have made this book an exceptional effort. Their encouragement from time to time has been an inspiration for everyone.

The publisher and the editorial board hope that this book will prove to be a valuable piece of knowledge for students, practitioners and scholars across the globe.

Index

www.ingramcontent.com/pod-product-compliance
Lightning Source LLC
Chambersburg PA
CBHW061945190326
41458CB00009B/2792